GASTRIC BAND HYPNOSIS EXTREME WEIGHT LOSS

Discover the Powerful Hypnotic Effect of Positive Affirmations.
Control Sugar Cravings and Weight Gain with
the Power of Meditation and Mindset Change

Table Of Contents

Introduction

T he Gastric Band is a hypnosis process used to change the lives of seriously overweight and obese people who've been unsuccessful at reducing weight using other techniques. It replaces the actual Gastric Bypass Surgery with a hypnosis-based different focused on achieving the very same result of reducing the quantity of food the stomach can take in one meal. While this sort of surgery of the mind is not new, its weight loss application is unique.

Researchers worldwide agree that one of the keys to wellness, health, and individual growth depends on understanding the mind/body connection.

Gastric band hypnosis is more secure and less pricey than having the equivalent surgery executed.

The hypnotic gastric band system changes the size of your stomach, but it also helps you get comfortable and enjoy healthier foods. Hypno-gastric banding is a healthier, longer-term, non-evasive option. Changing your body physically cannot give you long-term results, but you can enjoy healthier alternatives by tackling the main problem of over-eating.

Your body is a genuinely astonishing machine. It produces all the energy you use. It keeps your heart thumping and your lungs breathing two 4 hours every day. It does a lot from using only the food you eat, the air you inhale, and the energy it has put away in your body. Simultaneously it fixes and keeps up itself while never halting work.

When we fit your hypnotic gastric band, that fueling, fixing, and maintenance system keeps on working similarly as nature intends, however, there will be a couple of significant differences:

1. You will have less space for food in your stomach.

2. You will feel full sooner.

3. That "full" feeling will be urgent and easy to notice.

4. You are probably going to encounter changes in your food choices.

5. With the hypnotic band, there is no physical medical procedure, and therefore no physical dangers.

6. The hypnotic band is a less expensive

As you are eating less, your body might be pickier or search out new foods to guarantee it gets all the sustenance it requires. You don't need to stress over this with your conscious mind by any means. You keep on eating exactly what you need, but you'll see that what you need to eat changes. In the early stages, those progressions might be very subtle, so it might take you a little effort to understand that you currently find various foods more appealing.

The Magic of Your Digestive System

It will be useful to have a diagram of your digestive system with the goal that you see how your hypnotic gastric band functions. A few people are interested and keen on how the body functions; others are most certainly not. Notwithstanding, whatever you deliberately think, it is significant that you read this segment with the goal that your conscious mind has all the information it needs to process my hypnotic instructions. So regardless of whether you discover this segment somewhat complex, simply continue reading because your conscious mind will comprehend and use all it needs from this clarification.

Your digestive system begins functioning when you smell your food. Your salivary glands begin to secrete saliva when the food enters your mouth; saliva begins to blend in with it to make it simpler to swallow and to start to breakdown the diet. Next, the physical movement of chewing your food sends signals to your stomach to release hydrochloric acid. When you swallow, the food goes down your throat, or in medical terms, your esophagus. At the base of your throat is a solid valve called a sphincter, which unwinds to give the food access to your stomach. The sphincter shields your throat from the acid in your stomach. Sometimes, heartburn or overeating makes gastrointestinal reflux through that sphincter into your throat.

That builds up what we call indigestion. In your stomach, your food is blended in with acid and enzymes that break down the food into smaller particles. Proteins and fats take more time to process than sugars, so various foods take time to break down in the stomach. Vegetables do not take up to six0 minutes, and red meat can take a few hours to process. You don't need to worry about this, and your body does everything naturally.

From the stomach, your food, now broken down into micro pieces, is released bit by bit into your small intestine. Then, when the food goes into your intestines, your body extracts the nutrients for sustenance. Various enzymes further break it down into particles that are sufficiently small to pass through the walls of your intestines into the bloodstream. Carbohydrates are separated into glucose, which is taken to the liver. Glucose is used to control the muscles in your body. Proteins are separated into amino acids and sent into the bloodstream circulating all through the body and used to build and repair cells and tissues.

As the food goes through your small intestine, each of the nutrients is separated into various micro-molecules. In the colon, the water and salts that helped the process are absorbed once again into your body, and the rest is excreted. Every one of these processes is controlled by a lot of hormones, or signaling chemicals, in your body. In your digestive tract, one of the most important is called glucagon-like peptide-1 (known as glp-1). It is released as food enters your intestines. Glp-1 does loads of various jobs.

Since glp-1 does both these jobs at the same time, the feeling of fullness is connected to the process that gets energy into your muscles. This guarantees you don't feel full until your body is getting all the energy it needs. Levels of another hormone, called peptide yy (known as pyy), also increase when you have eaten. Pyy diminishes hunger and builds the capacity for nutrient absorption, so again it aids to signal you to stop eating to ensure you get what you need. Levels of a third hormone, called ghrelin, decline after a meal. Ghrelin is one of the hormones that cause us to feel hunger.

CHAPTER 1:

What it is Important to Know About Hypnosis

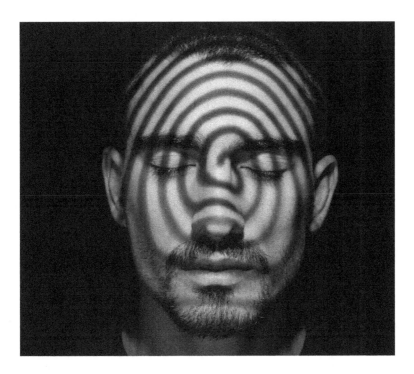

While brainwashing is a notable type of mind control that numerous individuals have about, hypnosis is additionally a significant sort that ought to be thought of. Generally, the individuals who know about hypnosis think about it from watching stage shows of members doing silly acts. While this is a sort of hypnosis, there is much more to it. This part is going to focus more on hypnosis as a type of mind control.

What Is Hypnosis?

To begin with, what is the meaning of hypnosis? As indicated by specialists, hypnosis is viewed as a condition of cognizance that includes the engaged consideration alongside the diminished fringe mindfulness that is described by the member's expanded ability to react to recommendations that are given. This implies the member will enter an alternate perspective and will be substantially more defenseless to following the recommendations that are given by the trance inducer.

It is broadly perceived that two hypothesis bunches help to depict what's going on during the hypnosis time frame. The first is the changing state hypothesis. The individuals who follow this hypothesis see that hypnosis resembles a daze or a perspective that is adjusted where the member will see that their mindfulness is, to some degree, not quite the same as what they would see in their common cognizant state. The other hypothesis is non-state speculations. The individuals who follow this hypothesis don't believe that the individuals who experience hypnosis are going into various conditions of awareness. Or maybe, the member is working with the subliminal specialist to enter a sort of inventive job authorization.

While in hypnosis, the member is thought to have more fixation and center that couples together with another capacity to focus on a particular memory or thought strongly. During this procedure, the member is likewise ready to shut out different sources that may be diverting to them. The mesmerizing subjects are thought to demonstrate an increased capacity to react to recommendations that are given to them, particularly when these proposals originate from the subliminal specialist. The procedure that is utilized to put the member into hypnosis is knitted hypnotic enlistment and will include a progression of proposals and guidelines that are utilized as a kind of warm-up.

There is a wide range of musings that are raised by specialists with regards to what the meaning of hypnosis is. The wide assortment of these definitions originates from the way that there are simply such huge numbers of various conditions that accompany hypnosis, and nobody individual has a similar encounter when they are experiencing it.

Some various perspectives and articulations have been made about hypnosis. A few people accept that hypnosis is genuine and are suspicious that the legislature and others around them will attempt to control their minds. Others don't have faith in hypnosis at all and feel that it is only skillful deception. No doubt, the possibility of hypnosis as mind control falls someplace in the center.

There are three phases of hypnosis that are perceived by the mental network. These three phases incorporate acceptance, recommendation, and defenselessness. Every one of them is critical to the hypnosis procedure and will be talked about further underneath.

Induction

The principal phase of hypnosis is induction. Before the member experiences the full hypnosis, they will be acquainted with the hypnotic enlistment method. For a long time, this was believed to be the strategy used to place the subject into their hypnotic stupor. However, that definition has changed some in current occasions. A portion of the non-state scholars has seen this stage somewhat in an unexpected way. Rather, they consider this to be the strategy to elevate the members' desires for what will occur, characterizing the job that they will play, standing out enough to be noticed to center the correct way, and any of the different advances that are required to lead the member into the correct heading for hypnosis.

There are a few induction procedures that can be utilized during hypnosis. The most notable and compelling strategies are Braid's "eye obsession" method or "Braidism." There are many varieties of this methodology, including the Stanford Hypnotic Susceptibility Scale

(SHSS). This scale is the most utilized instrument to examine in the field of hypnosis.

To utilize the Braid enlistment procedures, you should follow several means. The first is to take any object that you can find that is brilliant, for example, a watch case, and hold it between the centers, fore, and thumb fingers on the left hand. You will need to hold this item around 8-15 crawls from the eyes of the member. Hold the item someplace over the brow, so it creates a ton of strain on the eyelids and eyes during the procedure with the goal that the member can keep up a fixed gaze on the article consistently. The trance inducer should then disclose to the member that they should focus their eyes consistently on the article. The patient will likewise need to concentrate their mind on that specific item. They ought not to be permitted to consider different things or let their minds and eyes meander or, in all likelihood, the procedure won't be effective.

A little while later, the member's eyes will start to enlarge. With somewhat more time, the member will start to accept a wavy movement. If the member automatically shuts their eyelids when the center and forefingers of the correct hand are conveyed from the eyes to the item, at that point, they are in the stupor. If not, at that point, the member should start once more; make a point to tell the member that they are to permit their eyes to close once the fingers are conveyed in a comparable movement back towards the eyes once more. This will get the patient to go into the adjusted perspective that is knaps hypnosis.

While Braid remained by his method, he acknowledged that utilizing the acceptance procedure of hypnosis isn't constantly fundamental for each case. Analysts in current occasions have typically discovered that the acceptance strategy isn't as essential with the impacts of hypnotic recommendation as recently suspected. After some time, different other options and varieties of the first hypnotic acceptance procedure have been created, even though the Braid strategy is as yet thought about the best.

Recommendation

Present-day sleep induction utilizes a variety of proposal shapes to be fruitful, for example, representations, implications, roundabout or non-verbal recommendations, direct verbal proposals, and different metaphors and recommendations that are non-verbal. A portion of the non-verbal proposals that might be utilized during the recommendation stage would incorporate physical manipulation, voice tonality, and mental symbolism.

One of the qualifications that are made in the kinds of recommendation that can be offered to the member incorporates those proposals that are conveyed with consent and those that progressively tyrant in the way.

Something that must be considered concerning hypnosis is the contrast between the oblivious and the cognizant mind. There are a few trance specialists who see the phase of the proposal as a method of conveying that is generally guided to the cognizant mind of the subject. Others in the field will see it the other way; they see the correspondence happening between the operator and the subconscious or oblivious mind.

They accepted that the recommendations were being tended to directly to the conscious piece of the subject's mind, as opposed to the oblivious part. Braid goes further and characterizes the demonstration of trance induction as the engaged consideration upon the proposal or the predominant thought. The fear of a great many people that subliminal specialists will have the option to get into their oblivious and cause them to do and think things outside their ability to control is inconceivable as per the individuals who follow this line of reasoning.

The idea of the mind has additionally been the determinant of the various originations about the recommendation. The individuals who accepted that the reactions given are through the oblivious mind, for example, on account of Milton Erickson, raise the instances of utilizing aberrant recommendations. Huge numbers of these aberrant proposals, for example, stories or representations, will shroud their expected importance to cover it from the cognizant mind of the subject. The subconscious recommendation is a type of hypnosis that depends on the hypothesis of the oblivious mind. If the oblivious mind was not being utilized in hypnosis, this sort of recommendation would not be conceivable. The contrasts between the two gatherings are genuinely simple to perceive; the individuals who accept that the recommendations will go fundamentally to the cognizant mind will utilize direct verbal guidelines and proposals, while the individuals who accept the proposals will go essentially to the oblivious mind will utilize stories and analogies with concealed implications.

In both of these hypotheses of figured, the member should have the option to concentrate on one article or thought. This permits them to be driven toward the path that is required to go into the hypnotic state. When the recommendation stage has been finished effectively, the member will, at that point, have the option to move into the third stage, powerlessness.

Powerlessness

After some time, it has been seen that individuals will respond contrastingly to hypnosis. A few people find that they can fall into a hypnotic stupor reasonably effectively and don't need to invest a lot of energy into the procedure by any means. Others may find that they can get into the hypnotic daze, however, simply after a drawn-out timeframe and with some exertion. Still, others will find that they can't get into the hypnotic stupor, and significantly after proceeding with endeavors, won't arrive at their objectives. One thing that specialists have discovered intriguing about the weakness of various members is that this factor stays steady. If you have had the option to get into a hypnotic perspective effectively, you are probably going to be a similar path for an incredible remainder. Then again, if you have consistently experienced issues in arriving at the hypnotic state and have never been entranced, at that point, almost certainly, you never will.

There have been a few distinct models created after some time to attempt to decide the defenselessness of members to hypnosis. A portion of the more established profundity scales attempted to construe which level of a daze the member was in through the discernible signs that were accessible. These would incorporate things, for example, unconstrained amnesia. A portion of the more present-day scales works to quantify the level of self-assessed or watched responsiveness to the particular recommendation tests that are given, for example, the immediate proposals of unbending arm nature.

As per the examination that has been finished by Deirdre Barrett, there are two kinds of subjects that are considered profoundly vulnerable to the impacts of subliminal therapy. These two gatherings incorporate dissociates and fantasizers. The fantasizers will score high on the assimilation scales, will have the option to effortlessly shut out the boosts of this present reality without the utilization of hypnosis, invest a great deal of their energy wandering off in fantasy land, had fanciful companions when they were a youngster, and experienced childhood in a situation where nonexistent play was energized.

CHAPTER 2:

How to Transform Your Mindset

Our minds are very strong tools in our lives. How we behave and react to situations is a result of our mental conditioning and thought process. For a person to transform a certain behavior, for instance, quitting smoking or kicking an addiction to electronic devices, the transformation must start in mind first. What we instill in our subconscious minds is want we portray outside. For instance, if you are overweight due to overeating or eating the wrong kinds of foods, there may be underlying issues to your behavior. To transform your behavior, you must begin by transforming your mind. By use of hypnosis, a person can transform their mind and achieve their desired change.

Using Hypnosis to Transform Your Mind

The idea of hypnotherapy brings out reactions ranging from "cross-arm and wary in dismay" to "shocked in unadulterated amazement and surprise." There is no denying the supernatural quality encompassing spellbinding; it stays to puzzle individuals' psyches around the world.

As a result, we tend to live our lives amid a society in which the day to day rush of events doesn't leave us much time for thought and contemplation. This means that we are faced with making difficult choices in terms of dealing with our happiness and wellbeing.

Fortunately, this idea is a long way from a reality of true to life when you grasp spellbinding. In this way, we have a greatly improved idea.

What about utilizing the incredible intensity of hypnotherapy rather than manufacturing a universe of a completely perfect world?

Since there is a persuading reason for hypnotherapy behind the cloak of wizardry and visual impairment, to fix our brains, bodies, and in the long run, our universe.

As a general rule, trance has been utilized worldwide as an instrument for mending for in any event 4,000 years; however, science has just begun to exhume this entrancing riddle in most recent years. Their outcomes hugely affect our ability to change our thoughts and convictions, conduct, and practices, just as our recognition and reality to improve things.

In any case, most importantly, science has discovered a solid reality: entrancing is valid. What's more, on the off chance that you accept you've never had mesmerizing, accept again.

Hypnosis' characterizing practices are:

Increased suggestibility. Making musings progressively open and responsive.

Improved creative thinking. Creation in the eye of our psyches of striking, frequently illusory symbolism.

Without thinking, discernment. Quieting the cognizant systems that create thoughts while improving passionate mindfulness.

These 3 characterizing highlights make spellbinding a particular and effective instrument for private transformation.

A large portion of the issues that unleash destruction on the globe today happen because we have significant mental wounds to which there has been no inclination.

We download information from the globe around us at lightning speed until we're around 9 years of age. During this minute, our subliminal feelings and practices are normally shaped — before we built up our balanced reasoning (got when our mind frames the prefrontal cortex).

In our childhood, for instance, someone can let us know, "you're ugly." At the time, our brains can't defend the likelihood that any individual who reveals to us this will have a poor day or experience the ill effects of their psychological wounds. Rather, our energetic, honest personalities accept, "goodness, I'm frightful." That works for "you're stunning" on a kinder note, just as some other great attestation.

We are important making machines in this incredibly porous minute in our life. We quickly credit importance to them when certain events happen in our youthfulness. What produces our subliminal convictions is that allotted significance.

This is the place hypnotherapy comes in. Nothing fixes these significantly established enthusiastic wounds more rapidly than the hypnotherapy prescription. We have discovered that, in the condition of mesmerizing, we can get to and interface legitimately with these intuitive zones of our psyche—without our normal cognizant reasoning.

During trance, a trance inducer controls their patients back to their youth's zenith occasions. The patient can reassign centrality to them once recollections of the case reach them.

Reprogramming Your Mind through Hypnosis

Your intuitive personality has an enormous impact in dealing with your background—from the sorts of sustenance you eat to the exercises you take each day, the income level you get, and even how you react to unpleasant conditions.

Your intuitive feelings and understandings manage all of it. In a nutshell, your subliminal personality resembles an airplane's auto-pilot work. Following a particular way has been pre-modified, and you cannot go astray from that course except if you initially change the customized guidelines.

The "intuitive" is your mind's part that works underneath your customary arousing cognizance level. At this moment, you are primarily utilizing your cognizant personality to peruse these expressions and retain their centrality. However, your subliminal personality works hectically in the background, engrossing or dismissing information dependent on a present perspective on the globe around you. When you were a tyke, this present observation began to shape. Your intuitive personality drenches like wipe data with each experience.

While you were youthful, your consciousness rejected nothing since you had no prior perspectives that would negate what it saw. It simply recognized that it was genuine every one of the information you acquired during your initial puberty. You can almost certainly observe why this sometime down the road turns into an issue. Each time you were called by somebody stupid, useless, slow, apathetic, or more terrible, your subliminal personality put away the information for reference.

You may likewise have messages about your life potential or requirements relying upon your physical aptitudes, the shade of the skin, sex, or money related status. By the minute you were 7 or 8 years of age, you had a solid premise of religious on all the programming you viewed from people in your lives, network shows, and other natural impacts.

Since you are developed, you may figure you can simply dispose of the destructive or false messages you've consumed in your initial life. However, it isn't so basic. Keep in mind this information is put away underneath your cognizant awareness level. The main minute you understand this is the point at which it constrains your advancement in building up an actual existence that is adjusted, prosperous, and gainful.

Have you, at any point, endeavored to arrive at a target and consistently undermined yourself? Goading, right? It is fundamental to comprehend that regardless of what you do, you are not flawed or destined to come up short. You are bound to have some old, customized messages that contention with the new conditions that you need to make.

This is incredible news since it suggests that on the off chance that you first set aside the effort to reconstruct your intuitive personality, you can achieve pretty much anything! Before we discover how to reconstruct your psyche, it's fundamental to comprehend that the programming proceeds right up 'til today. You draw certain discoveries with each experience you have and store the messages that will direct your future conduct.

Procedures to Reprogram Your Mind

There are numerous particular techniques to overwrite your psyche mind's constrained or hurtful messages.

You could work with every one of these methodologies simultaneously; however, on the off chance that you pick only a couple of procedures to start, it will be significantly more effective. Rather than skipping around and weakening your endeavors, you need to give them complete consideration. Keep in mind; additional strategies can generally be consolidated after some time.

Impacts From the Environment Around You

Have you, at any point, respected your psyche mind's effect on your setting? Keep in mind that your subliminal personality is always engrossing information and reaching determinations dependent on that information and framing convictions.

Envision what sorts of messages are being ingested into your psyche if your day by day condition is loaded up with cynicism and struggle. Your first meditation is to carefully limit from this time on the antagonism to which you are oppressed. Except if you thoroughly need to watch the news and avoid investing a lot of energy with' lethal' people.

Rather, search for helpful information to peruse and watch, and burn through the vast majority of your minute with people who are sure and effective. You will locate that all the more reassuring messages are retained in your brain after some time, which will change how you see yourself and your potential.

Representation

Your subliminal personality responds well to pictures. Representation is an amazing method to utilize ideal, incredible pictures to program your brain. Attempt to picture advantageous scenes that element you and your background for 10–15 minutes every day.

Here are a few things you should envision:

- Fulfilling connections

- Passionate work

- An exquisite home extraordinary excursion

Whatever else you need to bring into your lives. As you do this always, you wind up redrawing the unfavorable pictures put away from your past encounters, concerns, concerns, and questions. Make sure to emanate incredible, positive emotions as you picture these excellent things in your brain to further expand the quality of representation. Permit love, satisfaction, appreciation, and harmony to move through you as though you truly had these encounters.

The message will be consumed by your subliminal personality, as though it were real! This is the genuine excellence of perception—the expert to sidestep confining messages and focuses on wonderful pictures that are altogether retained into your subliminal to replay later.

Affirmations

Affirmations are another effective method to place positive messages into your intuitive.

On the off chance that you observe a couple of straightforward standards, they work best:

- **Positively word them in the current state**. Declare "I'm certain and fruitful" rather than "I will be sure and effective," because are concentrating on a future condition doesn't compute with your intuitive personality — it just comprehends this time. Utilize helpful articulations too. Saying "I am not a disappointment" is determined as "I am a disappointment" since it is incomprehensible for your intuitive to process negative things.

- **Call for the proper feelings**. Saying "I am rich" while feeling poor just sends your subliminal clashing messages. Whatever words you state right now, attempt to feel the sentiments because your intuitive will be bound to think it.

- **Repeat, reiteration, redundancy**. On the off chance that you simply state it on more than one occasion, certifications don't work. Discuss them for the most elevated results ordinarily during the day. The decent thing about this is you can reveal to yourself attestations, so they can accommodate your routine flawlessly.

The Excitement of the Brain Through Binaural Beats

Another regular procedure is to utilize sound chronicles that purposefully change the recurrence of your brainwaves. It might seem like something from a sci-fi film. However, records are overwhelmingly positive from people who have endeavored these sound projects.

Contingent upon what you're doing at any predefined minute, your brainwaves fall into a particular recurrence:

- Gamma when you're engaged with certain motor capacities

- Beta when you're completely mindful and effectively centering

- Alpha when you've loosened up, Theta when you're lazy or languid.

- Delta when you are in significant rest

"Binaural beats" lead when two tones are performed at particular frequencies, causing an unmistakable example in your brainwaves. For example, you tune in to a sound that causes the alpha state if you needed to move from worried to lose. These sound projects can help reconstruct your subliminal personality by building up a progressively responsive gathering for advantageous messages to be introduced.

Research has demonstrated that when you are extremely loose, as in the alpha or theta expresses, your intuitive personality is increasingly open to new information. Utilizing cerebrum preparing sound projects alongside insistences or perception can be a solid blend because your subliminal personality enables its protections to assimilate any message you need to program in promptly.

Simply unwind and focus on good pictures!

CHAPTER 3:

Emotional Eating and How Overcoming Emotional Barriers

What Is Emotional Eating?

People usually eat to beat physical hunger. However, some people are relying on food as a source of comfort or to address their negative emotions. Some also use food as a reward whenever they achieve their goals or when celebrating special events like birthdays or weddings. When you use food as a cover or a solution for extreme emotions, then you suffer from emotional eating. The feelings that trigger your eating are mostly negative, for example, stress, loneliness, sadness, or when you are grieving. However, it is not only the negative emotions that can cause emotional eating; some positive emotions such as happiness or feelings of comfort can also trigger emotional eating.

There is a difference in the way people use food to address their emotions. While some people rely on food when they are in the middle of their life situations, others may find comfort in food soon after the situation is over. They use food as a recovery tool. A problem associated with emotional eating is that it may prevent you from utilizing other adaptive approaches to problems. You should also know that emotional eating does not solve the issues you are going through. If anything, it only serves to make you feel worse. After eating, the original emotional problem remains unsolved, and on top of it, you find yourself feeling guilty about overeating. It is, therefore, essential for you to identify the problem of emotional eating and to take timely appropriate measures to stop it.

How to Recognize Emotional Eating

The best way for you to know if you are suffering from emotional eating is to find out whether you always eat because you are hungry or you eat impulsively. You should pay attention to your emotions and how you usually cope with them. Find out if you are utilizing food just for hunger or you are unconsciously overeating.

Once you are sure you have an emotional eating problem, take appropriate steps to stop it. This is because not all the food you eat is healthy. You will occasionally find yourself eating unhealthy food such as junk food and sweets, which could be detrimental to your health.

Common Features of Emotional Hunger

It is easy for you to mistake emotional hunger for normal physical hunger. You, therefore, need to learn how to make a distinction between the two forms of hunger. The following are some of the hints you can use to tell the difference between the two kinds of hunger:

Emotional Hunger Comes Unexpectedly

You tend to experience emotional hunger suddenly. The feelings of craving will then overwhelm you, forcing you to look for food urgently. On the other hand, feelings of physical hunger tend to grow gradually. Also, when you are physically hungry, you will not be overwhelmed suddenly by hunger, not unless you have gone for days without food.

Emotional Hunger Desires for Some Specific Food

If you are physically hungry, any food is right for you. Physical hunger is not too selective on the type of food to consume. You will feel satisfied eating healthy food like fruits and vegetables. On the other hand, emotional hunger tends to be selective on the food to consume. In most cases, emotional hunger craves unhealthy foods, such as sweets, snacks, and junk food. The craving for these foods tends to be overwhelming and urgent. You may experience strong desires for such food as pizza or cheesecake, and you have no appetite for any other type of food.

Emotional Eating Lacks Concern for Consequences

If you are involved in emotional eating, then in most cases you find yourself eating without any concern about the consequences of overeating on your general wellbeing. You also eat without paying attention to the food you are consuming. You are not concerned about the quality of the food or its nutritional value. All you care about is the quantity of the food to satisfy your craving. Your goal will be to eat as much food as possible. On the other hand, when you are eating because of physical hunger, you will be conscious of the quality and the quantity of food you are consuming. You will be concern about the health benefits of the food you are eating. You will also choose to eat a very well-balanced diet, which will prevent your body from overeating junk foods.

Emotional Hunger Is Insatiable

If you are suffering from emotional eating, your hunger cannot be satisfied no matter the amount of food you have consumed. Hunger as a craving will refuse to get out of your mind. You will keep craving more and more food, and soon, you will find yourself eating continuously without a break. On the other hand, physical hunger is satisfied the moment your stomach is full. You may experience feelings of physical hunger only during specific times of the day. This could be the response of your body once you have conditioned it to receive food at times of the day.

Emotional Hunger Is Located on Your Mind

Unlike physical hunger, the craving for food originates from your mind. Emotional hunger involves the obsession originating from your mind on some specific type of food. You find yourself unable to ignore or overcome this obsession. You then give in to it and reach for your favorite food.

On the other hand, physical hunger originates from the stomach. You feel the hunger pang from your stomach. You can also occasionally feel growling from your belly whenever you are hungry.

Emotional Hunger Comes with Guilt and Regrets

When you are suffering from emotional eating, deep down, you know your eating does not come with any nutritional benefits. You will then have feelings of guilt or even shame. You know you are doing your health a lot of harm, and you may start regretting your actions. On the other hand, physical eating involves eating to satisfy your hunger. You will not suffer any feelings of shame or guilt for meeting your bodily needs.

Causes of Your Emotional Eating

For you to succeed in putting a stop to your emotional eating habits, you need to find out what triggers them. Find out the exact situations, feelings, or places that make you feel like eating whenever you are exposed. Below are some of the common causes of emotional eating:

Stress

One symptom of stress is hunger. You tend to experience the feeling of hunger whenever you are stressed. When you are stressed, your body responds by producing a stress hormone known as Cortisol. When this hormone is produced in high quantities, it will trigger a craving for foods that are salty or sugary in nature as well as any fried food. These are the food which gives you a lot of instant energy and pleasure.

If you do not control stress in your life, you will always be seeking relief in unhealthy food.

Boredom

You could be eating to relieve yourself of boredom. You can also resort to eating to beat idleness. Besides, you may be using food to occupy your time because you do not have much to do. Food can also fill your void and momentarily distract you from the hidden feelings of directionless and dissatisfaction with yourself. Whenever you feel purposeless, you tend to reach out for food to make you feel better. However, the truth is that food can never be a solution to any of your negative emotions.

Childhood Habits

Emotional eating could be a result of your childhood habits. For example, if your parents used to reward your good behaviors with foods such as sweets, ice cream, or pizza, you may have carried these habits to your adulthood. You will find yourself rewarding yourself with your childhood snack whenever you accomplish a given task. You can also be unconsciously eating because of the nostalgic feelings of your childhood. This happens when you always cherish the delicacies you used to eat in your childhood. Food can also serve as a powerful reminder of your most cherished childhood memories, for example, if you were eating cookies with your dad during your outings together. Whenever you miss your dad, your first instinct is to reach out for the cookies.

Social Influences

Occasionally, you may need to go out with your friends and have a good time. During such outings, you can share a meal to relieve stress. However, such social events can lead to overeating. You can find yourself overeating at the nudge of your close friends or family encourages you to go for an extra serving. It is easy to fall into their temptation.

Avoiding Emotions

You may use eating as a way of temporarily avoiding the emotions you are feeling, such as the feeling of anxiety, shame, resentment, or anger. Eating is a perfect way to prevent negative distractions, albeit temporarily.

Habits and Practices, You Can Use to Overcome Emotional Eating to Lose Weight

Practice Healthy Lifestyle Habits

You will handle life's shortcomings better when you are physically strong, happy, and well-rested. However, if you are exhausted, any stressful situation you encounter will trigger the craving for food. In this regard, you need to make physical exercise part of your daily routine. You also need to have enough time to sleep to feel rested. Moreover, engage yourself in social activities with others. Create time for outings with family or close friends.

Practice Mindfulness by Eating Slowly

When you eat to satisfy your feelings rather than your stomach, you tend to eat so fast and mindlessly that you fail to savor the taste or texture of your food. However, when you slow down and take a moment to savor every bite, you will be less likely to indulge in overeating. Slowing down also helps you to enjoy your food better.

Accept All Your Feelings

Emotional eating is often triggered by feelings of helplessness over your emotions. You lack the courage to handle your feelings head-on, so you seek refuge in food. However, you need to be mindful of your feelings. Learn to overcome your emotions by accepting them. Once you do this, you regain the courage to handle any feelings that triggers your emotional eating.

Take a Moment Before Giving in to Your Cravings

Typically, emotional eating is sudden and mindless. It takes you by surprise, and often you may feel powerless in stopping the urge to eat. However, you can control the sudden urges to reach for food if you take a moment of 5 minutes before you give in. This allows you a moment to reconsider your decisions and eventually get the craving out of your mind.

Find Other Alternative Solutions to Your Emotion

Actively look for other solutions to address your feelings other than eating. For example, whenever you feel lonely, instead of eating, reach out for your phone and call that person who always puts a smile on your face. Look for good alternatives to food that you can rely on to feel emotionally fulfilled. If you feel anxious, learn to do exercises.

CHAPTER 4:

Change Bad Eating Habits Through Hypnosis

You realize you need to quit eating; however, you basically can't. You know you've had enough burgers to last you for the following three meals, yet you just can't resist the urge to keep on crunching ceaselessly as though your life relied upon it. You realize that you need to battle it, yet you can't make sense of how to end binge eating. It will be a long stretch; however, the uplifting news is there are ways on the most proficient method to stop binge eating, and these cures are necessarily inside yourself discipline's scope.

Binge or emotional eating is the propensity to the gorge to adapt to negative sentiments or stress; for example, when cutoff times are closer or remaining burden is accumulating as far as possible. Studies point to low self-regard as the most well-known reason for binge eating. Different variables incorporate the absence of help from family or companions, stress, and weight. People with weight issues tend to eat considerably more when they are emotionally upset, and when they start, they get lost about how to end binge eating.

In the USA alone, there are about 1.9 million individuals, or one out of 142 people has a binge eating issue. This sickness rises above sex and age. Step-by-step instructions to end binge eating is, for the most part, about building up the conviction to quit overeating NOW, before other wellbeing confusions begin springing up on you.

There's no compelling reason to feel lost anyway because here are some basic strides on the most proficient method to end binge eating that you can follow.

1. The initial step on the best way to end binge eating is to search for the clinical help of a therapist or a specialist who can capably set up your treatment, an endless supply of turmoil.

2. After seeing your primary care physician, ensure that you adhere to your treatment plan. There are different treatments that experts use with the goal that patients can control their inordinate yearnings for nourishment. Well, known medicines are psychological, social therapy, relational psychotherapy, and the utilization of antidepressants to counter the inclination to indulge in emotional pressure. The specialists are there to control the patient. However, the achievement principally lies on the patient.

3. Uncover those smothered sentiments to the specialist. The propensity for overeating didn't happen medium-term. There may be encounters or injuries that have made you take comfort from nourishment. Closure binge eating might be quicker if the specialist comprehends what these underlying feelings and meetings are, so the individual in question can help you outline good strive after nourishment and emotional learning.

4. Leave your storage room. Since it's a sickness, it is something that you ought not to mind your own business. There are a great many others out there who are having some issues with you are. The most effective method to end implies connecting with whatever care groups are accessible inside your range.

5. Converse with your primary care physician about changing your way of life to return you to good shape of stable living.

The most effective method to end binge eating requires solid self-discipline. Besides, depending on nourishment, you might need to take up different exercises to alleviate you when you are in an emotional session. Attempt yoga and various types of activities, or just connect with a companion or a care group at whatever point the urge comes up.

It has been seen that binge eating is progressively frequent in creating western nations and has been expanding in recent years. That is why you don't need to feel that you are distant from everyone else. There are many different ways that you can turn to the most proficient method to end binge eating. Recollect this is a problematic issue and ought not to be trifled with or be embarrassed about.

Significantly, you begin revamping a stable relationship with yourself to defeat the binge eating issues. It's certainly something that requires some investment to do, but on the other hand, it's the most significant relationship you have, and it must be supported.

Having a stable and positive relationship with yourself is significant. All things considered, how would you part with affection if you can't cherish yourself? If you have a respectable love for yourself, continue doing something that will continuously raise it to another level. A superior level. If you have been binge eating for quite a while and have discovered that your self-love simply isn't there, attempt a portion of these tips to improve the relationship and love for yourself. We ought to never abandon ourselves and on beating binge eating issues.

To manufacture a superior relationship with yourself and discover self-love progressively, attempt these eight hints:

1. Set solid limits. Figure out how to state no when you would prefer not to accomplish something, need more time, or are excessively worried about everything else going on in your life. You need to focus on yourself, and it's significant that you have limits, so the possibility to binge eat isn't as definite.

2. Find a workable pace. At the point when you invest energy alone, you will find such a large number of things about yourself that may have covered up for quite a while.

3. Practice positive self-talk. Negative emotions can outdo you and cause you to feel awful. Envision gorging without beating yourself up. Envision not permitting yourself to have any liable sentiments or self-contempt about the binge. Envision not being at the most reduced level conceivable. Consider what solid self-talk can accomplish for you and the closure of the battle with binge eating issues. Giving up and pushing ahead can genuinely turn your life around!

4. Figure out how to excuse. Absolution is something that can be difficult to do. Now and again, it can appear as though holding resentment bodes well. At the point when you hold resentment, your emotions stifle the development that is required to develop as an individual.

6. Show your feelings. It is anything but a solid plan to hold your opinions in. Instead, it's ideal for letting whatever emotion you are learning about come! Show your displeasure, bliss, or pity. Letting your actual feelings show you will yet be another positive development of not gorging.

7. Be consistent with yourself. Rather than continually beating yourself down, why not begin to laud the beneficial things that are going on in your life? Begin being compatible with yourself by indicating support for new ideas and adulating what you have just practiced.

8. No more flawlessness: Just act naturally. Quit attempting to be a person or thing that you are most certainly not! Show your real nature and be glad for the individual you have become throughout everyday life. Praise who you are by doing whatever it takes not to be great. There's nothing of the sort, and you'll never arrive at that objective. Permit yourself to be you simply!

The Real Issue with Emotional Eating

The issue with emotional eating isn't that we eat in light of feelings. If that were the situation, the arrangement would be as straightforward as finding an interruption in a snapshot of extraordinary sentiments. The thought is that if you occupy yourself, you will abstain from gorging. The center turns into a break rather than managing your feeling.

The main problem with emotional eating is our fear of permitting our feelings a chance to surface. What is so terrifying about feelings? In our quest for having a place and fear of being condemned, we stifle sentiments that we know don't think about what is going on in reality. They appear unexpectedly and don't address us in a natural language that we can react to without much effort. Like a youngster that won't quit annoying until they get what they need, sentiments divert us from keeping an eye on what needs to do. The battle between our feelings and keenness drain us of vitality and take steps to toss us into a wild emotional typhoon. Imagine a scenario where we can't bring ourselves back. What is the benefit of recognizing feelings that would freely humiliate us? We accept that if we acknowledge our sentiments, we would need to follow up on them. Our activities may, for all time, harm our own and expert connections. We would be marked emotional and nonsensical, prompting the most exceedingly awful destiny an individual can persevere estrangement.

So, we control our feelings by returning them where they have a place in our bodies. We conceal our sentiments and continue to act in what we see to be adequate conduct. Our notoriety stays unblemished, and connections endure one more near calamity. Until our bodies make some noise and state "enough." The possibility that feelings are damaging and that the agony is deplorable is the main thrust behind the motivation to stifle our inclination at any expense. Similarly, as we endeavor to occupy a youngster amidst a hissy fit with sweets, we divert ourselves with nourishment.

Consider the possibility that sentiments got middle of the road. Imagine a scenario in which we had confidence that our feelings would vanish as fast as they showed up all alone. Imagine a situation where we regarded feelings as a significant aspect of the human condition. Imagine a situation in which we could simply be with them without blame or disgrace. Would we need an interruption? Would there be a requirement for emotional eating?

Behind the entirety of life's poor decisions is fear. At the point when we surrender to fear and search for self-defensive instruments, we damage our ideal experience of life. We limit our development potential and further harm our self-regard.

Weight loss training works by creating a protected spot where fearlessness and self-certainty are the stages from which decisions are made. When you decide to take part in the chance of permitting yourself to be trained, you will learn procedures that will empower you to grasp your feelings instead of stifling them. By recognizing emotions, you will recover control and praise the totality of what your identity is. You will let loose vitality recently devoured by the inward clash and direct it towards satisfying your fantasies.

CHAPTER 5:

Build a Healthy Relationship with Food

Would it be advisable for you to start a better eating routine or create smart dieting propensities to get in shape? For some individuals, the main thing they consider with regards to weight reduction is that they ought to start eating better. In all actuality, for long-haul benefits, the propensity for eating nutritiously is a vastly improved alternative for a few reasons.

The very notice of "starting a better eating routine" infers that you will later fall off of that diet. That in that spot reveals to you that eating fewer carbs is a momentary way to deal with a way of life issue. Sure, craze diets may work for the time being, yet over the long haul, they, for the most part, don't give any genuine advantage. Individuals need to shed pounds and keep it off. By learning the best possible strategies for weight control and keeping up smart dieting propensities, you are substantially more liable to reach and remain at your ideal weight. Giving exceptionally nutritious foods in the best possible sums is the ideal approach to fuel your body and control your weight.

Many "prevailing fashion eats less" increase momentary fame for the straightforward explanation that they give present moment, quick weight reduction, these eating regimens are frequently founded on taking out some nutritious foods and supplanting them with shakes, caffeinated drinks or other enchantment elixirs, diet pills, high fiber blends or costly prepared dinners. Some of the time, definitely diminishing your calories is a piece of these weight control plans. It is imperative to recollect that your body is powered by the nourishment you eat. So as to work at an elevated level, be solid and enthusiastic, it is indispensable to supply your body with exceptionally nutritious foods. Expelling nutritious foods from your eating regimen in a hurry to get more fit can't insightful choice. At times quick weight reduction can accomplish more mischief than anything.

A great many people comprehend that your body's digestion is imperative to weight control. Think about your digestion as your degree of vitality use. Utilizing less energy can prompt weight gain, since muscle to fat ratio is an abundance vitality that gets put away in fat cells. By diminishing weight too quickly it can really make your body hinder your digestion. This, thus, can make you sleepover weight after the underlying quick weight reduction of an eating routine. Known as the yo-yo impact, this is a main source of disappointment for people hoping to get thinner and keep it off. By joining appropriate dietary patterns and reasonable exercise, you can successfully keep up your digestion working at its legitimate level, which will help with controlling your weight. Muscle-fortifying activity, which straightforwardly expands your digestion, is significant, as is normal cardio aerobic exercise.

A couple of key focuses on appropriate eating ought to be remembered. Eating a few generally little estimated dinners and snacks for the duration of the day is a superior methodology than bigger, less continuous suppers. Try not to skip breakfast - it truly is the most significant dinner of the day. Eating normally keeps up your digestion. Select crisp foods and genuine items, including natural food sources, are vastly improved nourishment decisions than exceptionally handled, substance, and sodium-filled foods.

Numerous individuals believe that eating nutritiously is hard to achieve. The methodology one should take is to create good dieting propensities to get in shape, keep up legitimate weight, and augment your wellbeing. Propensities, both great and awful, are difficult to break. When you set up great dietary patterns, those propensities will be generally simple to keep up for the basic season; your eating techniques are only that - a propensity. Some portion of building up a decent nourishing project is figuring out how to basic food items look for good nourishment decisions. Most visits to the market lead you to similar paths and choosing similar nourishment things. By becoming accustomed to continually purchasing a choice of sound, nutritious foods, it will guarantee that you have these things in your home.

Another misinterpretation about appropriate eating is that nutritious foods are exhausting, tasteless, and not delicious. Nothing can be further from reality. Legitimate nourishment arrangement, cooking techniques, nutritious plans, and sound nourishment substitution can prompt some amazingly solid and delectable dishes.

With the best possible disposition towards your wholesome propensities, it very well may be enjoyment, sound, and scrumptious approach to legitimate weight control. The feared "starting a better eating routine" approach can stay away from as you create smart dieting designs on your approach to great wellbeing and legitimate weight reduction. In the event that you really record what you are eating regularly, you presumably will drop your jaw with sickening apprehension. We never think to include the little tidy portion size piece of candy here and the two treats to really observe the significant effect it is having on our weight control plans. The ideal approach to accomplish a solid way of life, to the extent our weight control plans go, is eating more products of the soil. We as a whole know it, so for what reason do we head for the potato chips aisle in the supermarket rather than the produce segment?

Essentially it comes down to this. Low-quality foods trigger our craving and leave us aching for additional. Ever wonder why eating one minimal honest Cheez-it prompts eating a large portion of a case? One taste triggers your body to need to continue eating. Presently in the event that you could condition yourself to do that with red grapes, we could accomplish that solid way of life. It might be hard to do, however, not feasible. Here are 5 different ways to condition yourself to settle on more beneficial nibble decisions.

Smart Dieting Ha Portions #1: Out of Sight, Out of Mind

On the off chance that you don't have shoddy nourishment in your kitchen, you won't eat it. It truly is that straightforward. I am the sort of individual who needs something to eat while I watch my daily film, and I will, in general, get the terrible stuff. The main occasions I don't is the point at which I cannot. Do your shopping for food directly after you have eaten an enormous supper so you won't be eager for awful foods, yet rather great food sources. Leave the store with no low-quality nourishment yet with plenty of products of the soil. Your satchel and your tummy will thank you over the long haul.

Good Dieting Ha Portions #2: Add Fruits and Vegetables to Your Dishes

Some of the time, it is difficult to plunk down with a couple of strawberries without the chocolate plunge; you desire something terrible. That is the trigger nourishment shouting to you; however, you need not answer. Cut the strawberries up and add them to a bowl of oat. Toss in a couple of blueberries and raisins. Simply make sure to utilize skim milk and keep the sugar in the cabinet. Organic product has enough normal sweetness without anyone else. Consider it characteristic treats.

When was the last time you got amped up for eating carrot and celery sticks without plunging sauce? Likely never, yet that doesn't mean you never will. Add them to a little serving of mixed greens when you need a tidy portion. No, you cannot suffocate it all in greasy blue cheddar dressing.

That is a similar thing as plunge, is it not? A tad of vinaigrette dressing is the thing that your psyche ought to consider.

Good Dieting Ha Portions #3: Make a Compromise

In the event that you are following the American Diet, your palette presently pines for high salt and high-sugar foods. Stopping is never fruitful when it is done immediately. Individuals think they have to stop all the awful stuff at the same time, and afterward 3 days after the fact they wear out and return to negative behavior patterns. Being sound can't pass up the foods you love.

On the off chance that you need pizza, eat a cat with a bowl of natural product serving of mixed greens rather than French fries. In the event that you need Cheeze-Its, eat a bunch with a bunch of grapes rather than a large portion of the cheez-It box. Straightforwardness into it and gradually improve your dietary patterns.

Good Dieting Ha Portions #4: Load up on Liquids

Commonly we mistake strive after thirst. You think you are starving until you drink a decent reviving glass of water. At that point, your stomach feels somewhat fuller, and you have not included more calories in your midsection line. On the off chance that you make sure to drink fluids on a regular basis, you probably get yourself not in any event, thinking you are eager any longer.

So, in light of that, whenever you fear to request an excess of fettuccine Alfredo at your preferred Italian eatery, drink a tall glass of water before you request. You may want to pass that for a pleasant fresh plate of mixed greens with shrimp or chicken.

Smart Dieting Ha Portions #5: Take A Supplement

Once in a while, we get going in our lives and may have the best expectations to eat healthily; however, we cannot generally find solid foods to eat. Most candy machines don't offer carrot and celery sticks, shockingly. One route around this is to take a day by day supplement that gives all of you the sustenance you would get on the off chance that you ate heaps of products of the soil. This doesn't mean you should take them and keep eating giggles bars throughout the day, as you may have guessed. Garbage is still garbage.

Eating foods grown from the ground may not be something you are utilized to, however simply like whatever else, it takes some becoming accustomed to. Utilize the tips above to make progress simpler, yet don't take on a similar mindset as a con artist. Con artists never succeed, and in the event that it was simple, everybody would stroll around in very good shape. Carrying on with a sound way of life implies settling on solid decisions. The more you do it, the more benefits you will be.

CHAPTER 6:

Program Your Mind to Slim Your Body

Your mind holds the key to your life. You can either let your mind drive you to happiness or malcontent. The good news is that you have the power to reprogram your subconscious mind to lead the life you desire. When you were younger, your mind was a blank slate; it did not have any existing ideas, beliefs, or interpretation of events. Every time someone said something to you, the subconscious absorbed it and stored it away for reference. For example, if you were called fat, worthless, ugly, embarrassing, all that negative information stored away because the mind is always listening and always impartial.

Now that you are older and know better, you believe that it is merely a matter of getting rid of the false notions that your subconscious took hold of in your childhood and youth. It is easier said than done because the subconscious does not respond to the conscious mind. This is because your programming makes decisions for you. Take, for instance; you start a workout routine or a new diet. Your old programming reverts you to your old habits, and you fail miserably at your set goals. This habit can annoy and frustrate you, almost forcing you to abandon the quest for a healthier lifestyle. Before you embark on programming your mind to your slim body, keep in mind that you are already that person that you intend to become. You need to develop the capacity to find them within yourself. To learn how to reprogram your mind successfully, you must:

Make A Decision

Decide on the exact outcome you wish for yourself. With clarity comes the power to shape your subconscious in the new paths to follow. Once you have settled on what you want for yourself at this moment and in the future, you are offering your mind resources toward the fulfillment of your objectives. Write it down.

Let's say you want to be 17-pounds lighter by summer three months away. That is a clear-cut objective which you have set for yourself. Put it down clearly on paper, place it within sight so you can see it as often as possible. Therefore when "external" forces try to sway you to say, indulging or binge eating, you remember that you have set a goal. You have decided to shed seventeen pounds in three months. All of your mental power is aligned to help you accomplish this task.

Commit

Once you have made a clear decision, commit to sticking by it. Commitment means allowing the decision to inform your choices. You may, however, expect to encounter fear. Fear is the biggest threat to success. The fear of failure drives people into giving up on their dreams- not failure itself. Fear can lead to procrastination of your goals, which in turn feed the fear with negative thoughts such as, "I am better off not trying" or "Why should I risk disappointment in case I fail?" These thoughts cause you to feel even worse than you did before. The best solution for fear is facing it.

Failure is not the end of everything; it is a lesson in itself. Access the first trial, everything you did, and how you did it. Examine if there is a way to modify the exercise to alter the result. Therefore, fear should not hold you back from your goals. Your efforts should be coupled with a commitment to a healthier lifestyle, devotion to overcoming the negative thoughts, and above all, commitment to yourself.

Modify Progress

Allow flexibility in your mental capacity. When you have committed to your decision, check the progress to see what is working and what can be amended. Striking a balance between alteration and overhaul can be difficult if you do not have a guide-be it a plan or a mentor or sponsor.

Do not limit yourself to the "It's my way or the highway" mentality. Having a peripheral vision can direct you to alternative possibilities and opportunities in case problems arise during your course. Adjusting your programming to cater to these speed bumps builds your resilience to challenges. Your subconscious develops a winning attitude where failures become lessons, hurdles become catapults, and change becomes inevitable.

Reprogramming Your Mind to Overcome Limitations

To overcome limiting beliefs, you must first acknowledge them and accept them for what they are and the role they have played in your life to this crucial point. The reason it is of significant importance to accept them is that you cannot change what does not exist. These beliefs are repeated to us by society, causing us to relate negatively with ourselves, with food, money, and others. When you realize that these beliefs do not define your worth, you will start to see your true potential and develop self-confidence in your abilities. You will feel free to win at everything you set your mind.

Note Down Your Personal Limiting Beliefs

While getting rid of all your limitations, write down the beliefs that you have had from childhood that simply do not serve your purpose anymore. For example, "I am overweight" or "I do not look as good as my petite friends." Such beliefs have likely caused you to look upon yourself with disdain. The negative "I am" thoughts are not honestly what you think of yourself unless someone said them to you.

Understand Causality

The circumstances you find yourself in are not the cause of your limiting beliefs, but the effect. Let us take an example of struggling with weight; the reason you are "struggling" is because of your limiting beliefs about food and yourself. Knowing this, you can alter your mentality about your limitations and flip them to work for you instead of against you.

Along with learning how to reprogram our mind, it is essential to note that the subconscious is still taking in new information and using it for reference for future decisions. There are several ways to reprogram your mind successfully.

Change Your Environment

The environment that surrounds us impresses significantly on our minds. Imagine if you always have people talking down at you at work or school. That kind of negativity can lead to a host of psychological problems, including depression.

Remove yourself from toxic environments; the instance you start to notice a pattern of ill-intentioned thoughts. Immerse yourself in an environment that fosters loving and positive thoughts. This way, your mind will absorb all the kind thoughts and gradually begin to reprogram your thought pattern. Support groups are an excellent environment to immerse yourself in because not only are these people working with the same set of circumstances, but some have also succeeded in daily progress. They know how rough it can be; therefore, they are the best reference for guidance and support.

Visualization

Visualization is a powerful reprogramming tool. Try to envision your transformed self in day-to-day activities. Envision your perfect romantic life, professional life, family relationships, financial relationships, as well as how you relate to yourself. See yourself as you would like to lead your life and allow yourself to feel fulfilled in these visions.

When these images are accompanied by emotions of accomplishment, gratitude, and joy, the more effectively they will redraw on your previous images. Your subconscious will see these images as the truth and will guide your decisions based on the repetitive visualization of the images.

For creative visualization to work, you must first change the underlying negative beliefs. This is because the subconscious, being the autopilot, corrects the shift in course whenever you seem to deviate from the norm. Ignoring the limiting beliefs can, by all means, curtail your efforts at reaching your objectives. Address the underlying cause first, or use the mental by-product focus method to attain what you want. This method allows you to focus on something that you do not have negative thoughts about, and therefore, by association helps you achieve what you desire. For example, you may want to travel abroad for summer vacation. You have been saving up for this trip, and you are looking forward to it. Visualizing your perfect self in your ideal trip will enable you to take the necessary steps to shred the undesired 17-pounds.

Help of Affirmations

Affirmations are necessary when you want to focus on another thought pattern. During affirmations, you phrase your statements positively, attach personal meaning to them, and repeat them to yourself multiple times throughout the day. Corresponding emotion helps the subconscious to understand the statements and believe them as the new status quo.

At first, getting your conscious mind on board with affirmations that may seem far-fetched can be difficult. As time goes on, however, the power of these affirmations has taken root into your subconscious, and you start to believe them to be true even with your rational mind.

Fake It Until You Make It

This method builds your self-esteem. It works in the same manner as affirmations but uses actions instead of thoughts and words. While your conscious mind is busy judging you about your deceiving mannerisms, your subconscious is loyally picking up on all the subtle differences in thought and sensation as you fake your way to your desired objective.

Actively changing your behaviors causes a change in habits, and sooner or later, your entire narrative will change.

Help of Hypnosis

Hypnosis is another tool used to reprogram the mind where the hypnotherapist puts you in a state of complete relaxation and reaches into the subconscious mind. Afterward, messages of empowerment and self-reliance are delivered repetitively to the listener. Hypnosis is used to reprogram the self-defeating habits and thoughts that keep you from achieving your goals.

This technique uses creative metaphors, illustrations, and suggestions to rewire the brain. In the wake of hypnosis weight loss studies, women who participated in hypnosis lost twice as much weight as the women who merely watched what they ate. The research, however, is not enough to be conclusive.

The best way to effect hypnosis is to play the messages when you are retiring for the day. As you are about to fall asleep, play the hypnosis tape, and let it carry your mind forward. Doing this in your sleep is more effective because there are limited to no distractions of the conscious mind chatter. The subconscious, being the sponge, absorbs the new thought patterns and rewrites the societal limitations previously held.

All these modes of rewiring your mind are dominant, but how exactly do you know what to expect? What signs do you look for to show improvement before you start discouraging yourself with negative thoughts? In short, when a paradigm shift takes place in your subconscious, you begin to feel a sense of change in your inner and outer self.

Training your mind is much more efficient than using mere willpower to weight loss. Only by repetitive insertion of positivity into the subconscious can new thoughts and habits become ingrained and manifest on the conscious level. To program your mind to become slimmer is not only about combating the eating habits but a general lifestyle approach that focuses on a healthier life that traverses beyond weight.

CHAPTER 7:

Weight Loss Meditation

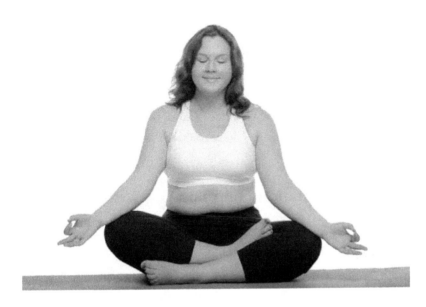

As we all know, meditation requires sitting still or even lying still. It doesn't sound like the sort of 'exercise' that'll help us lose weight, does it? How can meditation help you lose weight? Astonishing as it may be, weight loss meditation - in particular, 'meaningful meditation' - is increasingly being used by people who want to control the cravings of food and manage overeating. Often, diligent therapy may be used to reduce stress, thereby avoiding the 'comfort eating' arising out of stress. As we become more aware, we become more mindful of our cravings and can learn to pay attention to their underlying emotions, i.e., we can make a more informed decision before simply reaching for that sinful chocolate bar! When you continue feeding conscientiously every day so you will learn to like your food more over time, you'll now be more able to tell when you're full-meaning you'll continue eating fewer calories, of course. It has also been shown that consistent practice of mindful meditation lowers the stress hormone cortical. This is excellent news because high levels of cortical can cause pre-diabetes and central obesity (related to heart disease). In fact, cortical begins a process in our brains that can also lead to elevated hunger and intense cravings.

Don't Multi-Task

Experts say multi-tasking is our biggest enemy of weight control. When practicing careful weight loss meditation, it is important to concentrate on the food and the food alone. A recent study published in the 'Psychological Research' newspaper found that people who watched television at dinner were more likely to over-eat because they found the meal boring.

How Does Meditation Help You Get Weight Loss?

The truth is meditation rewires your consciousness. Feeding consciously is the opposite of feeding mindlessly. Eating more slowly helps your stomach realize when it's full-sometimes the stomach can take up to twenty minutes to signal to the brain that it's full and you shouldn't be hungry anymore. When consuming a limited amount of food, you would actually consume fewer calories all day long, resulting in a healthy and stable weight loss. There are books and CDs available which can teach you meditation techniques to reduce the urge to eat compulsively. Such training guides will help you overcome the cycle of compulsive eating so you can stick to your diet no matter what stress-causing incidents occur in your life. If it takes you a while to see results, don't be discouraged. It can take quite a bit of time to retrain your mind, so you no longer feel the temptation to overeat or eat mindlessly, particularly if it has been a lifelong problem. If you are not getting the effects you expect from directed therapy after giving it a period of time, consider consulting a counselor who is skilled in correcting compulsive behavior. Breaking the stress-based eating process is vital for your ability to stay on a diet and keep weight off after you leave the diet as you will no longer respond to stress by consuming large amounts of calories in your lifetime.

Weight Reduction Hypnosis and Self-Hypnosis

The notion of weight loss using self-hypnosis is definitely fascinating and one that would be nice to believe in. Hypnosis and self-hypnosis are now being used for various purposes, and the theory is embraced by many as much as possible. Strictly speaking, nobody is saying that by hypnosis, as if by a miracle, you can't make pounds go down. No, hypnosis is intended to reprogram your subconscious mind, so you have different behaviors. After all, your actions have much to do with your weight, as well as many other physical health aspects. It doesn't seem so hard to believe.

"Hypnosis" is a relatively new word, coined in the 19th century on the basis of a man named Franz Mesmer (from whom we got the word "mesmerism," meaning basically the same as hypnosis). It means going into a highly suggestible trance state. In more modern years, scientists have established different waves of the brain that exist during those phases. Hypnosis was initially identified with stage hypnotists and magicians, who under hypnosis can induce people to do funny or weird stuff. However, it was also used for therapeutic purposes at the same time. It fits well with the emerging field of psychology, which stressed the subconscious mind's role in our behavior.

Using Weight Loss Hypnosis

If you were using hypnosis to lose weight, how would you go about it? Well, you might get to visit a qualified hypnotherapist. Compared to any type of traditional therapy, this would not be cheap, but it has the advantage of being fast-acting. Many hypnotherapists rely on showing you methods that you can do on your own, and you don't need to go back to them for appointments all the time. A further option is to consider one of the endless videos which will help you lose weight. These can be played at your leisure, but you are unable to play them while driving or doing anything where you need your full conscious attention. Since hypnosis's focus is on the mind, it is also up to you to discover the specific methods that function best. In other terms, you can do your research and find a healthy diet that suits your body (not all person diet works well).

The real aim of weight loss hypnosis is to enable you to do the things you need to do to lose weight without having to exert so much power of will. If your subconscious mind is more aligned with your conscious goals, there is less chance of you sabotaging yourself by cheating on your diet or dropping off your exercise program. It may sound strange or exotic to use hypnosis to lose weight, but it is really just another way to use your mind in a way that supports your goals. Perhaps not for all, but if the idea sounds appealing or at least interesting, you may want to look into some of the weight-loss possibilities of using hypnosis.

CHAPTER 8:

Self-Improvement with Hypnosis

H ypnosis is rewiring your brain to add or to change your daily routine starting from your basic instincts. This happens due to the fact that while you are in a hypnotic state you are more susceptible to suggestions by the person who put you in this state. In the case of self-hypnosis, the person who made you enter the trance of hypnotism is yourself. Thus, the only person who can give you suggestions that can change your attitude in this method is you and you alone.

Again, you must forget the misconception that hypnosis is like sleeping, because if it is, then it would be impossible to give autosuggestions to yourself. Try to think about it like being in a very vivid daydream where you are capable of controlling every aspect of the situation you are in. This gives you the ability to change anything that may bother and hinder you from achieving the best possible result. If you are able to pull it off properly, then the possibility of improving yourself after a constant practice of the method will just be a few steps away.

Career

People say that motivation is the key to improving your career. But no matter how you love your career, you must admit that there are aspects of your work that you really do not like doing. Even if it is a fact that you are good at the other tasks, there is that one duty that you dread. And every time you encounter this specific chore you seem to be slowed down and thus lessening your productivity at work. This is where self-hypnosis comes into play.

The first thing you need to do is find that task you do not like. In some cases there might be multiple of them depending on your personality and how you feel about your job. Now, try to look at why you do not like that task and do simple research on how to make the job a lot simpler. You can then start conditioning yourself to use the simple method every time you do the job.

After you are able to condition your state of mind to do the task, each time you encounter it will become the trigger for your trance and thus giving you the ability to perform it better. You will not be able to tell the difference since you will not mind it at all. However, your coworkers and superiors will definitely notice the change in your work style and in your productivity.

Family

It is easy to improve in a career. But to improve your relationship with your family can be a little trickier. Yet, self-hypnosis can still reprogram you to interact with your family members better by modifying how you react to the way they act. You will have the ability to adjust your way of thinking, depending on the situation. This then allows you to respond in the most positive way possible, no matter how dreadful the scenario may be. If you are in a fight with your husband/wife, for example, the normal reaction is to flare up and face fire with fire. The problem with this approach is it usually engulfs the entire relationship, which might eventually lead up to separation. Being in a hypnotic state in this instance then can help you think clearly and change the impulse of saying words without thinking them through. Anger will still be there, of course, that is the healthy way. But anger now under self-hypnosis can be channeled and stop being a raging inferno. You can turn it into a steady bonfire that can help you and your partner find common ground for whatever issue you are facing. The same applies with dealing with siblings or children. If you are able to condition your mind to think more rationally or to get into the perspective of others, then you can have better family/friends' relationships.

Health and Physical Activities

Losing weight can be the most common reason why people will use self-hypnosis in terms of health and physical activities. But this is just one part of it. Self-hypnosis can give you a lot more to improve this aspect of your life. It works the same way while working out.

Most people tend to give up their exercise program due to the exhaustion they think they can no longer take. But through self-hypnosis, you will be able to tell yourself that the exhaustion is lessened and thus allowing you to finish the entire routine. Keep in mind that your mind must never be conditioned to forget exhaustion, it must only not mind it until the end of the exercise. Forgetting it completely might lead you to not stopping to work out until your energy is depleted. It becomes counterproductive in this case.

Having a healthy diet can also be influenced by self-hypnosis. Conditioning your mind to avoid unhealthy food can be done. Thus, hypnosis will be triggered each you are tempted to eat a meal you are conditioned to consider as unhealthy. Your eating habit can change to benefit you to improve your overall health.

Mental, Emotional and Spiritual Needs

Since self-hypnosis deals directly with how you think, it is then no secret that it can greatly improve your mental, emotional and spiritual needs. A clear mind can give your brain the ability to have more rational thoughts. Rationality then leads to better decision making and easy absorption and retention of information you might need to improve your mental capacity. However, you must set your expectations; this does not work like magic that can turn you into a genius. The process takes time, depending on how far you want to go, how much you want to achieve. Thus, the effects will only be limited by how much you are able to condition your mind.

In terms of emotional needs, self-hypnosis cannot make you feel differently in certain situations. But it can condition you to take in each scenario a little lighter and make you deal with them better. Others think that getting rid of emotion can be the best course of action if you are truly able to rewire your brain. But they seem to forget that even though rational thinking is often influenced negatively by emotion, it is still necessary for you to decide on things basing on the common ethics and aesthetics of the real world. Self-hypnosis then can channel your emotion to work in a more positive way in terms of decision making and dealing with emotional hurdles and problems.

Spiritual need on the other hand is far easier to influence when it comes to doing self-hypnosis. As a matter of fact, most people with spiritual beliefs are able to do self-hypnosis each time they practice what they believe in. A deep prayer, for instance, is a way to self-hypnotize yourself to enter the trance to feel closer to a Divine existence. Chanting and meditation made by other religions also lead and have the same goal. Even the songs during a mass or praise and worship triggers self-hypnosis depending if the person allows them to do so.

Still, the improvements can only be achieved if you condition yourself that you are ready to accept them. The willingness to put an effort must also be there. Effortless hypnosis will only create the illusion that you are improving and thus will not give you the satisfaction of achieving your goal in reality.

How Hypnosis Can Help Resolve Childhood Issues

Another issue that hypnosis can help is those problems from our past. If you have had traumatic situations from your childhood days, then you may have issues in all areas of your adult life. Unresolved issues from your past can lead to anxiety and depression in your later years. Childhood trauma is dangerous because it can alter many things in the brain, both psychologically and chemically.

The most vital thing to remember about trauma from your childhood is that given a harmless and caring environment in which the child's vital needs for physical safety, importance, emotional security, and attention are met, the damage that trauma and abuse cause can be eased and relieved. Safe and dependable relationships are also a dynamic component in healing the effects of childhood trauma in adulthood and make an atmosphere in which the brain can safely start the process of recovery.

Pure Hypnoanalysis is the lone most effective method of treatment available in the world today for the resolution of phobias, anxiety, depression, fears, psychological and emotional problems/symptoms, and eating disorders. It is a highly advanced form of Hypnoanalysis (referred to as analytical hypnotherapy or hypnoanalysis). Hypnoanalysis, in its numerous forms, is practiced all over the world; this method of hypnotherapy can completely resolve the foundation of anxieties in the unconscious mind, leaving the individual free of their symptoms for life.

There is a deeper realism active at all times around us and inside us. This reality commands that we must come to this world to find happiness, and every so often that our inner child stands in our way. This is by no means intentional; however, it desires to reconcile wounds from the past or address damaging philosophies that were troubling to us as children.

So, to disengage the issues that upset us from earlier in our lives we have to find a way to bond with our internal child, we then need to assist in rebuilding this part of us, which in turn will help us to be rid of all that has been hindering us from moving on.

Connecting with your inner child may seem like something that may be hard or impossible to do especially since they may be a part that has long been buried. It is a fairly easy exercise to do and can even be done right now. You will need about 20 minutes to complete this exercise.

Here's what you do: find a quiet spot where you won't be disturbed and find a picture of you as a child if you think it may help.

Breathe in and loosen your clothing if you have to. Inhale deeply into your abdomen and exhale, repeat until you feel yourself getting relaxed; you may close your eyes and focus on getting less tense. Feel your forehead and head relax, let your face become relaxed, and relax your shoulders. Allow your body to be limp and loose while you breathe slowly. Keep breathing slowly as you let your entire tension float away.

Now slowly count from 10-0 in your mind and try to think of a place from your childhood. The image doesn't have to be crystal clear right now, but try to focus on exactly how you remember it and keep that image in mind. Imagine yourself as a child and imagine observing younger you; think about your clothes, expression, hair, etc. In your mind go and meet yourself, introduce yourself to you.

CHAPTER 9:

The Power of Visualization

Continual visualization directs your actions to reflect that of your mental image. This is why it is possible to acquire new skills with creative visualization. You can also use it to give yourself a new set of belief system. You only need to visualize yourself believing in the mental image you create without allowing any resistance into your visualization. You have to reprogram any negative and limiting beliefs if you are to achieve your goal. There are two main ways you can apply this kind of visualization in your life:

• Ensuring a healthy life and banishing bad habits

• Fostering strong relationships

• Manifesting financial abundance

Healthy Living and Banishing Bad Habits

Bad habits often start innocently; an overindulgence during a holiday season that you do not seem to break even when the holidays are over, perfectly normal social situations that slowly get you hooked to the bad behavior, peer pressure, or unhealthy lifestyles. It may be drinking, smoking, over-eating, drug abuse, or gambling. These are all bad habits that undermine any idea you have of making your body and mind healthy. However, to have and maintain a healthy mind you need to have a healthy and happy body.

a) Use Creative Visualization to Heal

The best you can do for yourself is to use creative visualization. With the help of visualization, it is easy to break off any bad habits in your life and acquire the kind of perfect and healthy life you have been dreaming of. Creative visualization can help you quit smoking, reduce drinking and eating, and return your body to better shape in no time.

Through creative visualization, a positive attitude towards improving health can easily be developed. You only need to imagine yourself in that perfect body and health you dream of, and you can easily make it into reality. According to researchers, they found out that an ill person is likely to change the situation by mentally picturing themselves combating their illness. Such action has been proven to reduce the severity of symptoms in a patient and improve their quality and length of life.

However, always remember that when it comes to treating your illness with creative visualization, you must use it with tested procedures and medicines. It is good to get the best professional care and advice to be able to take care of your medical problems fast and effectively. The power of creative thinking only hastens your recovery and enhances the effectiveness of conventional medicine and professional help. It increases your defense for battling any illness you may have.

The whole process of visualizing your well-being is a partnership between you, your doctor, and your body. It is the doctor who determines what is ailing you and begins the medical treatment process to heal your condition. It is up to you to take the information you get from your doctor on where the problem is and pass it to your body. Through creative visualization you get your body to work on the problem at the same time you are receiving conventional medication. This is a process that can easily help you combat any serious and minor illness you have. It involves adopting a positive outlook on your health to keep your immune system in top shape.

b) Use Creative Visualization to Build Strong Core Muscles

As you grow older, your muscles weaken, especially if you are not active. A sedentary life makes your joints calcify, and this often leads to osteoarthritis. When you are young and active, you may not think about the aches and pain of joint problems. However, when you get to your middle ages, these pains become more pronounced. What you need to do is to keep your muscles in good condition.

When using creative visualization, remember that it is impossible to build muscles simply by visualizing them. You need to get active if you want to develop your core muscles and be physically fit. Visualization helps to hasten the process and give you the motivation to keep your mind on the desired results and maintain it.

The benefits of toughening your core muscles can be realized through:

• Improved posture and less low back pain

• Toned muscles that prevent the occurrence of back injuries

• Enhanced physical performance

• Less muscle aches

• Better balance made possible by having lengthened legs

According to physiotherapists and Pilates, the kind of physical and visualization exercise you engage in should emphasize to your body and unconscious mind the importance of keeping your muscles strong and fit to benefit you in all of the above-mentioned areas. They believe that this technique is the key to developing core stability. This is where your abdominal wall, lower back, diaphragm, and pelvis are able to stabilize your body during movement.

How to Combine Physical Exercise with Creative Visualization

Step 1: Do abdominal bracing in a sitting position - Sit up in an alert and straight manner. While maintaining a steady breath, try pulling your navel inwards to touch your spine. It is not enough to imagine this procedure. You must carry it out.

Step 2: Channel energy to your muscles - As you hold your navel in, feel the muscles that are being employed in the process. While in this position and state of mind, visualize yourself directing energy into your muscles from within you.

Step 3: Hold the position - If you are a beginner, you can hold this position for a minimum of 30 seconds. However, the recommended time is five minutes. Always remember to keep breathing evenly.

As you continue with this exercise, you need to try to apply feelings of power, vibrant health, and motivation to your body. This makes it easy to get the inspiration to match your visualization to your physical workouts. However, this is a technique that only works for small toning cases. For an overall toning of your body muscles, you need proper exercising techniques you can combine with creative visualization. Furthermore, if you have an existing health problem, have your doctor check you up and get the relevant professional medication your body requires before you begin this exercise program.

c) Use Creative Visualization to Look After Your Heart

There are very many benefits you get when your heart is healthy. When you ensure your heart is in good condition, you increase your blood flow and the distribution of oxygen all through your body. This lets you enjoy:

• High energy levels and increased endurance

• Low blood pressure

• Reduced body fat and a healthier body weight

• Less stress, anxiety, and depression

• Better sleep

The best way to look after your heart is to engage in aerobics. This is an exercise that causes you to breathe deeply and makes you sweat for a minimum of 20 minutes. Whether it is fast walking, swimming, jogging, biking, or even cross-country skiing, you should be in a position to make a conversation.

How to Combine Aerobics with Creative Visualization

Step 1: Visualize your exercise activity – In your mind, visualize taking a 20-minute jog, fast walk or any other aerobic activity. You can visualize yourself wearing the right exercising clothes and suitable running shoes.

Step 2: Visualize yourself doing the activity – Here, you need to visualize how you feel in the training wear, how the running shoes fit your feet perfectly, the country lane or suburbs in which you are running through, and start the exercise. Feel the power and strength in your feet and envision your arms moving back and forth to the rhythm of your legs. Feel the strength in your body and maintain your balance in a relaxed and simple position.

Step 3: Visualize yourself keeping pace for 20 minutes – In your mind's eye you can make yourself realize that although you are getting tired, you are also energized and can well keep your pace until you are done. Imagine sweat building on your brow; you mop it away; your body feels supple and is moving easily to the finish line.

Step 4: Imagine the scenery – As you jog, imagine passing trees, houses, and you nod to people or wave at them. You should seem to enjoy the fact that they see you serious about your health. In your mind, breath in and out, feel the refreshing coolness of the cool air and how refreshing it is to your lungs.

Step 5: Finish your exercise – You should continue your visualization exercise until you see yourself finish it. See yourself slowing down and returning to a normal walking pace and how your body feels fit and healthy.

While this visualization is still fresh in your mind, plan to get yourself a jogging gear to do a 20 minutes aerobic exercise. After your first jog, you will realize it is easy if you visualize the whole process and act it out as you exercise. You can do this exercise three times a week or more if you can to maintain a healthy heart. Remember to consult your doctor if you have any health issues before you start any aerobic exercises. Additionally, if you feel the exercise is painful for you or you become short of breath, you should stop.

d) Use Creative Visualization to Build Stamina

For you to overcome all the challenges that come with changing bad habits, you need to have both mental and physical stamina. This keeps you going and provides you with the energy you need to overcome through the long haul. Your mental stamina helps you stick to your plans up to their completion. It is the physical stamina that provides you the energy you need to move your body through the whole process of your plans.

When using creative visualization to build your stamina, you need breathing exercises. These exercises not only help you increase your stamina but also provide your body with the endurance you need to complete any activity you are engaged in. With the Chi breathing exercise, your goal should be to relax your shoulders and chest by breathing deeply from within your abdomen.

• Hold your hands over your lower stomach and sit in an upright position

• Breathe deeply until you cannot draw in more air and then let it all out to the last gasp

• Repeat this action more than once

• Visualize yourself breathing in with your hands sucking the air down all the way to your torso and into them

• Visualize yourself exhaling with your hands pushing air back through your stomach

• Slowly take your time settling into a slow, steady, and comfortable rhythm

• Imagine the deep and continuing energy each breath you take brings to you

As you breathe in and out, you should feel your abdomen expanding and contracting and the breathing moving all the way to your pelvic area. Practicing this exercise regularly is a good way to increase your endurance energy levels and build on your stamina level.

CHAPTER 10:

What is Gastric Band Hypnosis

What Is a Gastric Band?

A gastric band is a silicone device that is commonly used to treat obesity.

The device is usually placed on the upper part of the stomach to decrease the amount of food you eat. While on the upper part of the stomach, the band makes a relatively smaller pouch that fills up quickly and slows the consumption rate.

The band works when you make healthy food options, reduce appetite, and limit food intake and volume.

You do not need to experience these challenges when there is a simple and less invasive approach to achieve the same results as in a surgical gastric band.

Hypnotic Gastric Band

It is a natural healthy eating tool that can help control your appetite and your portion sizes. In this sense, hypnosis plays a significant role in helping you lose weight without the risk that comes with surgery.

It is now in the public domain that dieting does not solve lifestyle challenges that require weight loss and management.

Temporary diet plans are less productive, while continuous methods are challenging to maintain. Notably, these plans deprive you of your favorite foods and are too restrictive.

Deep down, you may have a problem with your body weight, and perhaps diets have not worked for you so far.

If you wish to try something that will provide a definite edge, you need to control your cravings for food hypnotically. By reaching this point, it is clear that you have prepared to try hypnosis, which has proven results in aiding weight loss.

How Does Hypnotic Gastric Band Work?

Typically, the conscious mind is not as receptive to suggestions, for it frequently analyzes and critiques them.

Chiefly, the complex network in your brain has different interpretations of the world around you, and most probably, unhelpful and harmful thoughts may have worked their way into that network.

As a result, you automatically become susceptible to uncontrolled unconscious urges such as overeating and ignoring serious bodyweight concerns. The hypnotic gastric band helps you dampen and overcome these uncontrolled thoughts and believe in suggestions that play a significant role in helping you alter your behavior.

Powerful affirmations: A change in lifestyle is mandatory if you wish to have permanent weight loss or control. Powerful statements are vital in changing your lifestyle slowly and surely.

Therefore, you should diligently practice regular affirmations for weight loss to realize the dream of losing weight. Notably, weight control is a direct function of your lifestyle as you are solely responsible for your behavior. In other words, your weight is determined by your mental attitude, the rest you take, physical exertion, and manner and frequency of eating. Use effective weight loss affirmations as a way to initiate the measure from your mind.

For real, it is necessary to change your thinking; otherwise, no form of dieting will ever help. Weight loss affirmations are significant in your mind, for they make you feel comfortable in your desired weight.

You should also consider the affirmations' wording to ensure that you focus on the solution but not the problem. For instance, you should not say, "I am not that fat," for that is the problem. Instead, you should focus on the solution and include words such as "I am getting slimmer" or "I am losing weight daily."

Write down healthy weight affirmations or take a cue from the samples I will provide. Repeating them shows that you are determined and sure to take the bold step of living and looking at a fitter life.

I weigh _ pounds: This affirmation sets the desired weight in your mind, and as you repeat the words, you remind yourself about your destiny and measures that you need to take.

I will achieve the ideal weight to enhance my physical fitness: You embrace lighter weight and improve on physical activity.

I love healthy food, for they help me attain an ideal weight: It promotes healthy eating and craving for healthy food.

I ease digestion by chewing all the food properly to reach my ideal weight: The affirmation is perfect before every meal as it guides the rate and amount of consumption.

I control my weight through a combination of healthy eating and controlling my appetite and my portion sizes:

It is a good idea to repeat these affirmations, among others, especially in front of a mirror, to keep reminding your subconscious mind about your goals. Most importantly, these affirmations work best while meditating or in a trance state. This combination will do wonders in your weight loss endeavor.

Powerful Visualization: With a hypnotic gastric band, your imagination should control your subconscious mind and body as a whole.

Visualizing weight loss means making the image of how you want to be in your mind's eye. It is an excellent tool that triggers the subconscious mind to shape your body to match your mental image. If you visualize accordingly, you will achieve weight loss, improve how you look, and become more energetic. Notably, emotions and thoughts affect the body for better or for worse. Negative thinking, anger, fear, stress, and worry, hurt the body and lead to the production of toxins that adversely affect you. On the other hand, if you are happy, confident, and positive, you energize and strengthen the body.

Learning how to use your subconscious mind in visualization effectively is to your advantage. Besides, it is a mental diet that you should incorporate into your weight loss plan. Chiefly, the success of the hypnotic gastric band will be higher if you eat healthily in addition to affirmations and visualization.

Visualization is such a great tool in the journey of leaving overeating and emotional eating behind. The significance of display lies not in our physical body but in the feeling of overcoming obsessions and challenges with food, weight, perfect body or plagues, and restrictions that keep you on the dieting merry go round.

With the hypnotic gastric band, visualization is a simple process, and you can use these few tips for weight loss.

· Find frequent moments where you sit down for several minutes and quietly visualize your slim body. Ignore all doubts, worries, and negative thoughts and maintain focus on the image.

· Forget your current look and imagine a beautiful and slim you with the ideal weight. See how gorgeous you look in a swimming suit and tight clothing that you always want to wear.

· Visualize peers and family complimenting your slim body and looks. Just watch the whole scene as if it is real and happening now.

· Feel free to construct different versions of these instances or other physical roles, such as dancing or swimming. Visualize yourself hearing compliments from other people about your slim body and watch them as they admiringly glare at you.

· Make the images you create in your mind colorful, realistic, and alive. See yourself in each of these real and exciting scenes in the ideal weight.

Avoid words that may destroy the efforts you may have made and let only the thoughts of your ideal weight and shape into your mind. Powerful visualization works wonders when practiced in hypnosis, for it makes the mental image a possible reality.

CHAPTER 11:

How to Know if
Gastric Band Hypnosis Works for You

Hypnotherapy for weight loss, particularly for portion control, is great because it allows you to focus on creating a healthier version of yourself safely.

When gastric band fitted surgery gets recommended to people, usually because diets, weight loss supplements, and workout routines don't seem to work for them, they may become skeptical about getting the surgery done.

Nobody wants to undergo unnecessary surgery, and you shouldn't have to either. Just because you struggle to stick to a diet, workout routine, or lack motivation does not mean that an extreme procedure like surgery is the only option. In fact, thinking that it is the only option you have left, is crazy.

Some hypnotherapists suggest that diets don't work at all. Well, if you're motivated and find it easy to stick to a diet plan and workout routine, then you should be fine. However, if you're suffering from obesity or overweight and don't have the necessary drive and motivation needed, then you're likely to fail. When people find the courage and determination to recognize that they need to lose weight or actually push themselves to do it, but continuously fail, that's when they tend to give up.

Gastric band hypnotherapy uses relaxation techniques, which are designed to alter your way of thinking about the weight you need to lose, provides you a foundation to stand on and reach your goals, and also constantly reminds you of why you're indeed doing what you're doing. It is necessary to develop your way of thinking past where you're at in this current moment and evolve far beyond your expectations.

Diets are also more focused on temporary lifestyle changes rather than permanent and sustainable ones, which is why it isn't considered realistic at all. Unless you change your mind, you will always remain in a rut that involves first losing and then possibly gaining weight back repeatedly. Some may even throw in the towel completely.

Hypnotherapy for Different Types of Gastric Banding Types of Surgeries

There are three types of gastric banding surgeries that could be used during hypnotherapy. These include:

- Sleeve Gastrectomy

- Vertical Banded Gastroplasty

- Mixed Surgery (Restrictive and Malabsorptive)

Gastric banding surgeries are used for weight loss. Depending on what your goal is with this weight-loss method, you can choose which option works best for you. The great thing about hypnotherapy with gastric band firming surgery is that you can get similar results if you practice the session consistently.

During gastric banding surgery, the surgeon uses a laparoscopy technique that involves making small cuts in the stomach to place a silicone band around the top part of your stomach. This band is adjustable, leaving the stomach to form a pouch with an inch-wide outlet. After you've been banded in surgery your stomach can only hold one ounce of food at a time, which prevents you from eating more than you need to in one sitting. It also prevents you from getting hungry.

Given that it is an invasive procedure, most people don't opt for it as an option to lose weight. During the procedure, you are also placed under anesthesia, which always involves some risks. Nevertheless, the procedure has resulted in up to 45% of excess weight loss, which means that it can work for anyone looking to shed weight they are struggling to lose. The procedure can also be reversed should the patient not be happy with the effects thereof. When reversed, the stomach will return to the initial size it had before the surgery. (WebMD, n.d.)

Undergoing one of these three gastric banding surgeries, there are some side-effects involved, which include the risk of death. However, this is only found in one of every 3000 patients. Other than that, common problems post-surgery include nausea and vomiting, which can be reduced by simply having a surgeon adjust the tightness of the gastric band.

Minor surgical complications, including wound infections and risks for minor bleeding, only occur in 10% of patients. (WebMD, n.d.)

As opposed to gastric bypass surgery, gastric banding doesn't prevent your body from absorbing food whatsoever, which means that you won't have to worry about experiencing any vitamin or mineral loss in your body.

Types of Gastric Banding Techniques Used in Hypnotherapy for Weight Loss

• Sleeve Gastrectomy - This procedure involves physically removing half of a patient's stomach to leave behind space, which is usually the size of a banana. When this part of the stomach is taken out, it cannot be reversed. This may seem like one of the most extreme types of gastric band surgeries, and due to its level of extremity, it also presents a lot of risks. When the reasons why the sleeve Gastrectomy is done and gets reviewed, it may not seem worth it. However, it has become one of the most popular methods used in surgery, as a restrictive means of reducing a patient's appetite. It is particularly helpful to those who suffer from obesity. It has a high success rate with very few complications, according to medical practitioners. Those who have had the surgery have experienced losing up to 50% of their total weight, which is quite a lot for someone suffering from obesity. It is equally helpful to those who suffer from compulsive eating disorders, like binge eating. When you have the procedure done, your surgeon will make either a very large or a few small incisions in the abdomen. The physical recovery of this procedure may take up to six weeks. (WebMD, n.d.)

• Vertical banded Gastroplasty - This gastric band procedure, also known as VBG, involves the same band used during the sleeve Gastrectomy, which is placed around the stomach. The stomach is then stapled above the band to form a small pouch, which in some sense shrinks the stomach to produce the same effects. The procedure has been noted as a successful one to lose weight compared to many other types of weight-loss surgeries. Even though compared to the Sleeve Gastrectomy, it may seem like a less complicated surgery, it has a higher complication rate. That is why it is considered far less common. Until today, there are only 5% of bariatric surgeons perform this particular gastric band surgery. Nevertheless, it is known for producing results and can still be used in hypnotherapy to produce similar results without the complications.

• Mixed Surgery (Restrictive and Malabsorptive) - This type of gastric band surgery forms a crucial part of most types of weight-loss surgeries. It is more commonly referred to as gastric bypass and is done first, prior to other weight-loss surgeries. It also involves stapling the stomach and creates a shape of an intestine down the line of your stomach. This is done to ensure the patient consumes less food, referred to as restrictive mixed surgery, combined with Malabsorptive surgery, meaning to absorb less food in the body.

What You Need to Know About Hypnotic Gastric Band Therapy

If you're wondering whether gastric band surgery is right for you, you may want to consider getting the hypnotherapy version thereof. Hypnotherapy is the perfect alternative, it is 100% safe as opposed to surgery, which has many complications, and also a lot more affordable. It has a success rate of more than 90% in patients, which is why more people prefer it over gastric band surgery. Given that you can also conduct it in the comfort of your own home, you don't even have to worry about the cost involved. Overall it serves as a very convenient way to slim down, essentially shrinking your stomach.

Again, hypnosis doesn't involve any physical procedure involving surgery. It is a safe alternative that uses innovative and developed technology to help you get where you want to be. The hypnotherapy session involves visualizing a virtual gastric band being fitted around your stomach that allows you to have the same experience as you initially would during surgery, but without the discomfort, excessive costs, and inconvenience.

The effect is feeling as if you are hungry for longer periods, require less food, and experiencing a feeling of being full, even if you've only eaten half of your regular-sized portion. This will also help you make healthier choices and discover that you can indeed develop a much healthier relationship with food than you currently have.

If you're wondering whether gastric band hypnotherapy will work for you, you have to ask yourself whether you have the imagination to support your session. Now, of course, everybody has an imagination, but is yours reasonable enough?

If you can close your eyes and imagine yourself looking at something in front of you that is not there, and spend time focusing on it, then you can make it through gastric band hypnotherapy successfully.

It's normal to think before you start anything that if it isn't tailored to you specifically, it is likely to fail. However, visual gastric band hypnosis can offer you emotional healing. This supports your goals, including weight loss and health restoration. If you spend time engaging in it, you will learn that you can achieve whatever you set your intention on. You can remove your cravings subconsciously, eliminate any negative and emotional stress, as well as memories that form a part of your emotional eating pattern. Given that emotionality forms a big part of weight gain, you should know that it can be removed from your conscious mind through hypnotherapy and serve any individual willing to try it.

Gastric band hypnotherapy has a 95% success rate among patients, according to a clinical study conducted in the U.K. This study also proved that most people will be able to accept and succeed in hypnotherapy, but if they're not open to the experience, they won't find it helpful at all. People who are too closed off from new ideas, like hypnotherapy, which is often made out to be a negative practice among the uneducated, won't be able to relax properly for a hypnotherapist's words to take effect. (Engle, 2019)

After just one hypnotherapy session, you will know if it works, as it is supposed to start working after just one session. That is why hypnotherapy is not recommended for everyone. It's only suggested to anyone ready to change their feelings toward food. If you don't believe in it or that it will get you to where you want to go on your weight loss journey, it is deemed useless.

The cost of gastric band hypnotherapy sessions with a professional hypnotherapist can only be established after you've undergone an evaluation. Usually, every new patient requires up to five sessions in person. During these sessions, energy therapy techniques are also taught, which will help assist any struggle a patient may have with anxiety, anger, stress, and any other negative emotion.

CHAPTER 12:

Mind and Body Connection

People who experience disease, accidents and other trauma to their bodies often react by dissociating themselves from painful sensations and physical self-awareness. While this can be beneficial in the short term, it can also conflict with a person's ability to self-regulate and create meaningful behavioral improvements.

Obesity is a source of depression in itself, and weight loss consumers still detach from their bodies-this This is one explanation that they can over-eat and not be aware of actual satiation signals. When it comes to patterns and behaviors that may not benefit the development of well-being in general, parts of the body may respond negatively, given the individual's conscious intention to do otherwise.

Our mission is not only to teach customers about their mind-body connectivity, which happens to be bi-directional but to help them become more adept at using it as a healing tool. Because of this two-way function, we can take a "top-down" approach, change a person's way of thinking and feeling to affect changes in their physiology, or take a "bottom-up" tact physical functions to improve the thoughts and emotional state of a person.

Another approach I help clients work towards enhancing their awareness and responding to their bodies' signals and building self-acceptance is to use a massage on the abdomen. This strategy will also help overcome stomach issues that encourage unhealthy eating and drinking, or even traumatic conditions.

The abdomen is genuinely an energy source, a powerhouse in itself. The Japanese call this center of our body "hara," a place where "ki," or energy, is produced. During my martial arts training, I learned to embrace and focus on this part of my body, and once I did, I broke through some previous mental and physical limitations.

Releasing unhelpful discomfort in the abdomen can relax the entire body and mind, with several positive outcomes resulting:

1) Reduces chronic stress and anxiety and alleviates pain

2) Increases metabolism and enhances intestinal fires

3) Builds self-acceptance

4) Strengthens the connection between mind and body and increases awareness of physical sensations

Meditation for Mindful Hypnosis of the Heart

For individual communities like ours, people are admonished to "suck for your belly at a young age! "(Do you unintentionally keep stress in yours right now?!) Regardless of height and weight, we are full of self-awareness in this part of the body and feel inside. As a result, we are often detached from our heart and may have pessimistic feelings about it.

Even if a person doesn't struggle to be overweight, they can "keep" the gut unconsciously in a strengthened, restricted role. Practicing this belly exercise will make the enteric nervous system-the digestive tract-transition towards a "remembered health" more relaxed.

Sit quiet, with your eyes closed. Take your thoughts to the middle area, to your heart. Let yourself aware of how you feel about that part of your body. Let the emotions, concepts, and opinions rise into your consciousness, like bubbles flowing from the sea. Do not be your feelings; just watch them unfold. You can experience hearing your voice or hearing specific thoughts in someone else's voice as well. Just watch them as they float up.

You should count your breath as you breathe in, count as you catch your breath, and count as you breathe out. Using the diaphragm, you want to live heavily, and your abdomen inflates more than your chest region. It is a simple way to help the conscious mind shift away from disturbing or disruptive thoughts and activate relaxation. You might want to apply some imagery to it, including seeing a number written in sand and seeing a gentle wave wash it away, replacing it with the next number. And you can want to consider the numbers in your head.

Note when you do so that the stomach muscles are relaxed and other body muscles relax as they do. Just when your stomach settles, does it become possible to dissipate the pain in your body fades away? A surge of warmth passes over you and helps your mind to become calm, peaceful.

Then raise your right hand to the top of your uterus, gently resting it just below your bra line. Pressing gently in a clockwise direction, start rotating it to the left. It should rub your belly's outer circumference gently, reaching up to the tops of the arms, falling to the bottom of the navel, and then reversing the other hand. Your skin and flesh move by gentle pressure but will not feel uncomfortable.

Imagine that as you massage your "hara," you activate and balance the life-force within you. You link inside this personal, intense center. When you find that there are troubling thoughts or emotions, let them float both up and down. Consider that something that blocks, inhibits, or otherwise harms you is being dislodged and discharged.

Begin to breathe deeply and rhythmically, inhale excellent, soothing substances, and exhale all that isn't beneficial or curative. Imagine your healthy, fully working digestive tract, returned to optimal fitness. Bring in a state of peace, a state of well-being, just though you experience revitalization and regeneration of the energies within your heart.

When you've done 10-12 massage rotations, relax and indulge in the sensations of relaxation and calm now, realizing that you'll experience the good benefits of having this unique period as you return to your usual activities.

Spend a few minutes a day in abdominal yoga, and you will realize after a short time that not only the abdomen and overall body will feel better, but the digestive system will also change!

Body Parts

We may also use a method called "Body Parts" to enhance the connection between mind and body. This approach can be a stand-alone strategy, or it can quickly improve specific techniques you use to assist a customer. Ultimately, it acts as an excellent method to attract and expand a customer for future research. It helps to build hope that you will "open the door" between a person's aware and subconscious minds, encouraging them to connect openly to aspects of themselves that will be part of a "unit" of recovery.

Start with inducing some consumer concentration and relaxation. You can make them concentrate on breathing; they can place their attention on a hand or leg, leading them to close their eyes and finding they can still imagine that portion of their body, even with their eyes closed. The key goal is to focus their attention on their physical self.

Using something similar from here, like:

When you learn your side, now you may think about all the stuff the side does with you how it supports you in so many ways: touching, stroking, squeezing, grabbing, raising, folding, feeding (describing every client-relevant tasks)

A beautiful hand is a hand. I wonder if you should say what you think of what it does for you?

PAUSE

So, if the hand were able to talk, what would it tell you? And what is it you need?

PAUSE

That's right, and talk of your heart now, please the incredible pump the allows blood to circulate to keep you healthy. Your wonderful heart built to beat so many times in your lifetime. Nobody knows exactly how many cycles it is, but it works to achieve the beats for you. Who do you want your heart to tell?

PAUSE

So, what does the heart want to tell you about what it's going through about what you need? Hear it now.

PAUSE

That's right, and now just talk of your big toe on your left foot (* or some other, untouched part of your body, maybe an eyebrow or an ear)

That's helping you keep calm to make you walk. Your beautiful big toe builds to help you make more strides in your life.

No one knows precisely how many steps this is, but it works to do the number of moves for you. I'm curious if you will let yourself be overwhelmed with admiration of how good the toe works for you and will continue to.

PAUSE

So, would the toe like to talk to (any part of the body which needs healing) now? Should this happen, what will they tell each other?

PAUSE

Could you imagine pretend if you have to that all the well-being in that toe transmit in any way maybe even the code for that well-being can be replicated and pasted anywhere throughout the body it's needed now (provide patter explaining where and how it's required?

That's right, so now think about your lungs, those magnificent lungs that draw in and filter fresh oxygen for you to keep you healthy. The excellent lungs build to breathe in and out too many times in the lifetime. Well, no one knows just how many times it is, but they are trying to satisfy the number of breaths for you.

PAUSE

So, what do the lungs want to tell you what they're going through what they need from you?

I might recommend that a client needs a real chat about their knees and liver in any area of the body that has suffered through lifestyle decisions. I may even encourage the client to get support with their hands, who are often involved in poor eating habits, to function more closely towards their objectives.

Following these conversations, suggest that ALL parts of the body integrate, as part of the whole ... working together towards wellness, promoting comfort, balance, healing, continued enlightenment and improvement, etc.

* With a few tactics, we will put in a balanced body part:

1. In a diversion to the cycle from dealing with the negative side of being overweight or obese, it momentarily focuses away from what is wrong with the body.

2. As a resource for body parts that need healing.

Every part of the body is negatively affected by the extra weight and should approach it this way. Having room for an interactive conversation with a person and their body will provide them with knowledge, perspective, and inspiration and promote calming reactions within the body.

CHAPTER 13:

Gastric Band Hypnosis Training

The physical gastric band requires a surgical procedure that involves reducing the size of your stomach pocket to accommodate less volume of food and, as a result of the stretching of the walls of the stomach, send signals to the brain that you are filled and therefore need to stop eating any further.

The hypnotic gastric band also works in the same manner, although in this case the only surgical tools you will need are your mind and your body, and the great part is you can conduct the procedure yourself.

The hypnotic gastric band also conditions your mind and body to restrict excess consumption of food after very modest meals.

There are three specific differences between the surgical (physical) and hypnotic gastric bands:

- In using the hypnotic band, all necessary adjustments are made by continued use of trance.

- There is an absence of physical surgery and therefore you are exposed to no risks at all.

- When compared with the surgical gastric band, the hypnotic gastric band is a lot cheaper and easier to do.

How Hypnosis Improves Communication between Stomach and Brain

How would you know when you have had enough to eat? Initially, you will begin to feel the weight and area of the food. When your stomach is full, the food presses against and extends the stomach well, and the nerve endings in the walls of the stomach respond. When these nerves are stimulated, they transfer a signal to the brain, and we get the feeling of satiety.

And, as the stomach fills up and food enters the digestive tract, PYY and GLP-1 is released and trigger a feeling of satiety in the brain that additionally prompts us to quit eating.

Sadly, when individuals always overeat, they become desensitized to both the nerve signals and the neuropeptide signaling system. During the initial installation trance, we use hypnotic and images to re-sensitize the brain to these signs. Your hypnotic band restores the full effect of these nervous and neuropeptide messages. With the benefits of hypnotic in view, we can recalibrate this system and increase your sensitivity to these signs, so you feel full and truly satisfied when you have eaten enough to fill that little pouch at the top of your stomach.

A hypnotic gastric band causes your body to carry on precisely as if you have carried out a surgical operation. It contracts your stomach and adjusts the signals from your stomach to your brain, so you feel full rapidly. The hypnotic band uses a few uncommon attributes of hypnotic. As a matter of first importance, hypnotic permits us to talk to parts of the body and mind that are not under conscious control. Interestingly as it might appear, in a trance, we can really convince the body to carry on distinctively even though our conscious mind has no methods for coordinating that change.

The Power of the Gastric Band

A renowned and dramatic case of the power of hypnotic to influence our bodies directly is in the emergency treatment of burns. A few doctors have used hypnotic on many occasions to accelerate and improve the recuperating of extreme injuries and to help reduce the excruciating pains for their patients. If somebody is seriously burnt, there will be damage to the tissue, and the body reacts with inflammation. The patients are hypnotized to forestall the soreness. His patients heal quite rapidly and with less scarring.

There are a lot more instances of how the mind can directly and physically influence the body. We realize that chronic stress can cause stomach ulcers, and a psychological shock can turn somebody's hair to grey color overnight. In any case, what I especially like about this aspect of hypnotism is that it is an archived case of how the mind influences the body positively and medically. It will be somewhat of a miraculous event if the body can get into a hypnotic state that can cause significant physical changes in your body. Hypnotic trance without anyone else has a profound physiological effect. The most immediate effect is that subjects discover it deeply relaxing. Interestingly, the most widely recognized perception that my customers report after I have seen them—regardless of what we have been dealing with—is that their loved ones tell them they look more youthful.

Cybernetic Loop

Your brain and body are in constant correspondence in a cybernetic loop: they continually influence one another. As the mind unwinds in a trance, so too does the body. When the body unwinds, it feels good, and it sends that message to the brain, which thus feels healthier and unwinds much more. This procedure decreases stress and makes more energy accessible to the immune system of the body. It is essential to take note that the remedial effects of hypnotic don't require tricks or amnesia. For example, burns patients realize they have been burnt, so they don't need to deny the glaring evidence of how burnt parts of their bodies are. He essentially hypnotizes them and requests that they envision cool, comfortable sensations over the burnt area. That imaginative activity changes their body's response to the burns.

The enzymes that cause inflammation are not released, and accordingly, the burn doesn't advance to a more elevated level of damage, and there is reduced pain during the healing process.

By using hypnotic and imagery, a doctor can get his patients' bodies to do things that are totally outside their conscious control. Willpower won't make these sorts of changes, but the creative mind is more grounded than the will. By using hypnotic and imagery to talk to the conscious mind, we can have a physiological effect in as little as 20 minutes. In my work, I recently had another phenomenal idea of how hypnotic can accelerate the body's normal healing process. I worked with a soldier in the Special Forces who experienced extreme episodes of skin inflammation (eczema). He revealed to me that the quickest recuperation he had ever made from an eczema episode was six days. I realized that the way toward healing is a natural sequence of events carried out by various systems within the body, so I hypnotized him and, while in a trance, requested that his conscious mind follow precisely the same process that it regularly uses to heal his eczema, however, to do everything quicker.

One and a half days after, the eczema was gone. With hypnotic, we can enormously enhance the effect of the mind. When we fit your hypnotic gastric band, we are using the very same strategy of hypnotic correspondence to the conscious mind. We communicate to the brain with distinctive imagery, and the brain alters your body's responses, changing your physical response to food so your stomach is constricted, and you feel truly full after only a few.

What Makes the Hypnotic Work So Well?

A few people think that it's difficult to accept that trance and imagery can have such an extreme and ground-breaking effect. Some doctors were at first distrustful and accepted that his patients more likely than not had fewer burns than was written in their medical records, because the cures he effected had all the earmarks of being close to marvelous. It took quite a long while, and numerous exceptional remedies before such work were generally understood and acknowledged.

Once in a while, the cynic and the patient are the same individuals. We need the results, but we battle to accept that it truly will work. At the conscious level, our minds are very much aware of the contrast between what we imagine and physical reality. In any case, another astounding hypnotic marvel shows that it doesn't make a difference what we accept at the conscious level since trance permits our mind to react to a reality that is independent of what we deliberately think. This phenomenon is classified as "trance logic."

Trance logic was first recognized 50 years ago by a renowned researcher of hypnotic named Dr. Martin Orne, who worked for a long time at the University of Pennsylvania. Dr. Orne directed various tests that demonstrated that in hypnotic, individuals could carry on as though two absolutely opposing facts were valid simultaneously. In one study, he hypnotized a few people so they couldn't see a seat he put directly before them. Then he requested that they walk straight ahead. The subjects all swerved around the seat.

Notwithstanding, when examined regarding the chair, they reported there was nothing there. They couldn't see the seat. Some of them even denied that they had swerved by any means. They accepted they were telling the truth when they said they couldn't see the seat, but at another level, their bodies realized it was there and moved to abstain from hitting it.

The test showed that hypnotic permits the mind to work at the same time on two separate levels, accepting two isolated, opposing things. It is possible to be hypnotized and have a hypnotic gastric band fitted but then to "know" with your conscious mind that you don't have surgical scars and you don't have a physical gastric band embedded. Trance logic implies that a part of your mind can trust one thing, and another part can accept the direct opposite, and your mind and body can continue working, accepting that two unique things are valid. So, you will be capable to consciously realize that you have not paid a huge amount of dollars for a surgical process, but then at the deepest level of unconscious command, your body accepts that you have a gastric band and will act in like manner. Subsequently, your stomach is conditioned to signal "feeling full" to your brain after only a couple of mouthfuls. So, you feel satisfied, and you get to lose more weight.

Visualization Is Easier Than You Think

The hypnotic we use to make your gastric band uses "visualization" and "influence loaded imager." Visualization is the creation of pictures in your mind. We would all be able to do it. It is an interesting part of the reasoning. For instance, think about your front door and ask yourself which side the lock is on. To address that question, you see an image in your mind's eye. It doesn't make a difference at all how reasonable or bright the image is, it is only how your mind works, and you see as much as you have to see. Influence loaded imagery is the psychological term for genuinely significant pictures. In this process, we use pictures in the mind's eye that have emotional significance.

Although hypnotic recommendations are incredible, they are dramatically upgraded by ground-breaking images when we are communicating directly to the body. For instance, you will be unable to accelerate your heart just by telling it to beat faster. Still, if you envision remaining on a railroad line and seeing a train surging towards you, your heart accelerates pretty quickly. Your body overreacts to clear, meaningful pictures.

CHAPTER 14:

Weight Management Program

Well, there are some other effective ways in which an individual can lose weight. You might decide to combine them to make the processes faster and more manageable. What meditation does is that it will help you enhance some of these factors. You may find that the activities you chose to undertake become more effective as you conduct them. We do not disregard the methods; we only recommend that you complement them with meditation.

In some cases, you find that mediation can be useful on its own. While in other cases, you have to combine it with other activities to help an individual struggling with weight loss. We will go through some of the other things that you might need to look at as you get on a weight loss journey. Below are some of them.

Dieting

This is perhaps the first thing we think of any time we think of weight loss. We gain weight as a result of the poor eating habits that we adapt, and they cost us a lot. Eating wrong does not only make us add weight, but it can also affect our health.

We have some diseases that result from eating unhealthy foods. Plant-based meals tend to be nutritious and, at times, provide the best solution for weight loss. We shall discuss three weight-loss diets that an individual can utilize to lose weight.

Ketogenic Diet

A keto diet is a low carb diet. It utilizes the concept of consuming high fat and the required amount of proteins while also taking a low carb diet. Carbohydrates are mainly composed of sugars. When we increase their consumption, we have excess sugars in the bloodstream that cannot be converted into energy. In the process, your body converts it into fats, and you end up gaining weight. A keto diet helps an individual lose weight by lowering the intake of carbohydrates. You only consume what your body requires; hence, no sugar needs to be converted into fats. You find that while using this diet, you can also burn the excess fats in your body. This works in a process known as ketosis. When the intake of glucose and other sugars is low, the body begins to convert the fats in the body into energy. When this process occurs consistently, you can manage to get rid of all the excess fats, and as a result, you lose weight.

Paleo Diet

Its name was generated from the fact that it was the diet used during the Paleolithic era. If you have studied history, you probably know the events that occurred in this particular period. During such times, there were no processed foods, and people would eat vegetables, fruits, seeds, nuts, and meat. In that era, there was barely any obesity case since people ate what they planted or what they hunted. People came up with the ideology that if that type of diet helped people keep fit, then it can be an excellent diet to adapt to this era. Much of the weight gain is as a result of consuming food substances that are processed. They have no nutritious benefits to our bodies; instead, we drink a lot of food that has no use. We get full and satisfied after the meal, yet the body does not utilize the food. We end up gaining extra weight with no nutritious benefit. With the help of a Paleo diet, you get to consume that which you need. The body utilizes the food consumed to the maximum, and in the end, you keep fit and barely add extra weight.

Mediterranean Diet

The main inspiration behind a Mediterranean diet comes from the eating habits of the people living in the Mediterranean region. Some of the countries involved were Italy and Greece. Their menu was composed of fruits, unrefined cereals, vegetables, olive oil, and legumes. It also included some moderate consumption of meat, animal by-products, and wine. People using this diet were found to be healthy due to the nutrients contained in the food that they consumed. It was challenging to get diseases that result from poor eating habits. Lifestyle diseases were difficult to come by, especially this type of diet. The diet helps an individual lose weight since they get to take up what is required by the body. It also ensures that they maintain their weight. While taking this diet, you lower your carbohydrate intake. This means that you reduce the sugar levels in your bloodstream and that what you eat is what you require. Your body acquires the right amount of sugars, so there are no excess sugars that need to be converted into fats. That is how the Mediterranean diet helps you lose weight and have a healthy body.

How Does Meditation Help While Dieting?

You might be wondering how meditation can help while dieting and ensuring that you lose weight. Dieting can be difficult, especially if you are not disciplined enough to do so. You might find yourself having some regular cheat days, which may appear more recurrently than they should. You find that you are regularly doing this and end up not dieting at all. Meditation brings you into realizing some of the poor decisions that you make as far as eating is concerned. As a result, you can make better decisions once you understand where you went wrong. Dieting can be challenging, and you need to stay focused for you to manage to complete the diet successfully.

If you are dieting to lose weight, you need to observe the food every single day keenly. This is to help you ensure that the dieting will be useful in accomplishing its purpose. In the beginning, you will face a lot of temptations, but you can manage them with the aid of meditation. It ensures that you stay focused on the goal, and you manage to lose weight as planned.

Exercise

You might be the type of individual that immediately thinks of the gym anytime you hear about losing weight. You could believe that there is something that you physically need to do to cut off the weight. In the process, you might acquire a gym membership, and you set a gym routine whereby you get to go to the gym at certain times during the day. Even while exercising, you need meditation. Meditation allows you to concentrate on the various activities that you are undertaking. In the process, you get to give your full energy into the activities that you are taking. You find that even the various exercises that you engage in become useful in helping you lose weight. It allows you to burn the extra fats and maintains a good shape.

There is a lot of incredible power in meditation. In that calm state of mind, incredible things happen. It more like a magical occurrence. Your account becomes keen and focused on the things that matter. In the process, you find that your performance levels are increased as you make better decisions regarding the issues at hand. This may seem like an easy thing to do, but we barely do it. An individual may find the process of meditation tedious for them to handle, yet it requires a small amount of your time. At that moment, you get to relax your mind as you think of the conditions around you. During your gym time, as you are busy exercising, you can use some of that time to meditate. This will improve your concentration and can, at times, cause you to be energized. The process of exercising can get tiring, and you need to find a way to ease the burden that comes with it. With meditation, this is easily achievable.

Consuming the Necessary Amount of Food

At the time, we waste a lot of food that is not necessary. You only find that you eat because there is food to be consumed and not because you need it. With the help of meditation, there is a lot that you can accomplish. Eating when there is no need to can lead to weight gain. Your body keeps taking foods in excess quantities that it does not need. As this process progresses, you find yourself adding a lot of weight. Meditation will help you avoid some of these incidences by helping you make the right decisions. When it comes to eating, you only do so when it is necessary.

You can plan your meals and the amount you wish to consume at a given time in a day. For instance, during breakfast, you might decide to eat a heavy meal. This is to provide you with the strength that you need to tackle the day. Breakfast is an essential meal, so you are allowed to eat slightly more than the other meals. During lunchtime, you can eat a slightly smaller portion than that of breakfast.

On the other hand, at night, you can ensure that you take the smallest part. At night there is no significant activity to be carried out unless you are working a night shift. The recommended amount you should consume should be just enough to carry you through the night. In between the day, you can include some small snacks and ensure that they are healthy snacks. If you manage to follow this keenly, your weight loss journey will be effortless. Meditation will play a significant role in ensuring that you consume the amount of food that is necessary and according to your meal plan.

Healthy Eating Habits

There are certain habits that we adapt to, and that contributes to weight gain. For instance, you might have a habit of eating too fast, and as a result, food is not well processed. This causes the food to become waste, and instead of benefiting your body, it becomes a problem for your organization. In some situations, you might find that what you consumed had some nutritious benefits, but due to your poor eating habits, it does not help you in the way that it should. At times, you might cook a lot of food or even serve yourself a lot of food. You might get to a point whereby you feel like you are already full. However, you keep eating because there is food on your plate or because you have some leftover food. The excess food you consume once you are full will not help your body, so you can find yourself adding weight.

CHAPTER 15:

Gastric Band Techniques

Placing

In this meditation, you will learn how to walk along a beautiful beach walk, allowing you and deeply relax.

Follow me on this mental vacation as we place an emotional and mental, and gastric band around your stomach, which will allow you to feel full as soon as you eat exactly as much food as you need.

So, get into a comfortable seated position, on your favorite spot, so that you are undisturbed for the rest of this session. As you relax, the gastric band will become more powerful and influential over your life. Take a big deep breath, relax, and then exhale the tension and worry as you close your eyes. Feel your body already slowing down. Take another breath and let to go with a sigh of relief. This moment is for you to practice your new lifestyle, of being full, at the perfect time. Now say to you with faith, "overeating is impossible for me."

Now breathe into the truth of these words as you breathe them out into reality. You are creating a smaller stomach. Relax and breathe, and then use the power of your imagination to visualize a beautiful beach with white sand, reflecting in the sunlight. It looks like snow. You can see the turquoise waters fading to a deep blue as the ocean goes deeper.

Look down into the sand where you stand, and notice the beautiful bits of shells with all different colors and textures as you see dried seaweed scattered about something that catches your eye buried into the sand, it is your preferred color. So, as you get closer, you will see that it is a small yet thick band that is as big around as your fist, and it just so happens that it is the most vivid version of your favorite color. The brightness of this hue brings you joy. The curious, round band, flashing of your most beloved color choice is called the gastric band

It is placed around the top of your stomach, cinching down the amount your stomach can hold. So, it makes your stomach feel smaller, which gives you that feeling of fullness that you've had enough to eat. This band only exists in the medical world. But you can get the same results, using the power of your mind, by placing the band within and around your stomach in this relaxing session.

Feel your feet entering the sand and allow yourself on each step to relax more and more. Notice the powdery texture, dispersing under your feet, and allow it deeply soothe you. Feel the ocean breeze, and smell the salty air. As you walk, you will get tired. A perfect chair has appeared just for you, facing the ocean. So have a seat and recline backward with your gastric band in your hand. Familiarize yourself with its shape and size. It is like a small belt that can be tightened and loosened.

This relaxing gastric band session brings you to perfect health and weight through the power of your mind. It brings about a new and improved positive attitude to life with intention, positivity, and knowing when enough is enough. Now bring your hands into the mode of prayer and notice how you feel. Notice your mind and body going back on track, firmly ready to eat the healthy amount.

Take a few calming, relaxing moments before coming back to the present moment. Take a long breath in and feel the gastric band as it's limiting your ability to overeat. Feel the band affecting the weight throughout your body. When you are ready, just gently open your eyes. And then seal this in with a grateful smile.

Tightening

Welcome to this relaxing meditation. This meditation will guide you to a pristine lake that is surrounded by mountains and help you to tighten your gastric band, making for an even smaller stomach that will fill up quickly. Get yourself into a nice seated position where you can easily fully let go, and you will not be disturbed by the surrounding world.

As you get into a powerful state of relaxation, begin to imagine that you are tightening this gastric band, and as you do so, you will find that weight-loss becomes easier and easier by the day. Now begin to breathe deeply while allowing your body to expand. Exhale all of your stress out and take another deep breath in, and as you exhale and allow, let your eyes gently closed.

Now notice how you feel. Notice how your body is settling down and as it becomes relaxed as we go along. Let go of any current worries or obligations. Enjoying for yourself, and you begin your health and wellness journey from the first session by placing a gastric band near your stomach with the power of your mind. So, appreciate yourself for taking on this amazing opportunity.

Now say to yourself, "I will eat only as much food as I need. I need less food to feel full."

Breath in, and allow these words to become part of every level of your awareness. Breathe out any doubt and breathe in any truth that you are capable of eating just the right amount to have the perfect shape, size, and overall wellness. Now relax, calm down, and be at complete ease. Let your body slow down just a little bit more. Activate your imagination by bringing into your mind the eye, the site of a magnificent lake that is surrounded by mountains. And the sky, which is a crisp turquoise blue dappled with the cloud. And the sun is shining all around you. The waters of this lake are crystal clear, and it's reflecting the blueness of the sky. The water is acting as a mirror for the mountain range.

Now become aware of your stomach and notice it becoming smaller from your wonderful session on the beach when you first found your gastric band. Feel how your stomach is comfortable and happy about its new size and wants to become even smaller.

As you walk toward the lake, notice the soil under your feet, becoming smooth and supportive. As you go near to the water edge, dip your toes in the cool and fresh aqua. Even though your feet are submerged, the waters of this mystical lake relax your entire body.

Notice beside you the small red canoe waiting for you. Enter into this canoe and pick up the beautiful hand-carved oar. The oar signifies the ability to be able to tighten your gastric band. Dip the oar into the water, moving to the bottom of the lake, and push off the shore. Feel as this simple movement helps to tighten your gastric band by a millimeter.

Also, visualize yourself in your kitchen now preparing your next meal. You will find that when you put the plate on your food, all of your choices are healthy. You will notice that you will only scoop a small amount of each item because you have a good ability to put the right amount of food that you need on your plate, now with your gastric band supporting you. You don't want to waste a bite of food. You should only eat the perfect amount.

See yourself eating this healthy meal and shocked at the small food that it took for you to feel satisfied. Now, as you rise from this wonderful meditation, allow the image of the canoe and the see-through water to fade away from your mind, as well as the great mountains and along with the visual of your next meal.

Right now, bring yourself back from this experience into reality. Breathe in deeply, and become aware of your surroundings in the present moment. Wiggle around your toes and fingers a little bit and feel the fresh new energy and wisdom coming into you. And then, whenever you are ready, open your eyes.

Removal

So far, you have placed this band around your stomach while walking on the relaxing beach and tightening the band while rowing your canoe on a crystal-clear lake. Right now, we will visit an ancient Japanese castle to be able to remove this band and discard it during the beautiful ceremony. Now make sure that you're in a comfortable position, in a place that you can enjoy practicing this relaxing session. This is the final step in your gastric band experience. So, take a nice deep breath in and then breathe out while closing your eyes.

Relax your body. Feel it sinking into the chair or bed, soft and supportive underneath you.

Breathe in and then breathe out while noticing the gentle rise and fall of your chest as you breathe in. Now start becoming aware of your abdomen and feel how slim it is as you're, eating less food. You are becoming fuller and making hunger outdated. You know that you're supposed to eat, but eating doesn't consume your day or your mind. You only eat when you should eat and refuse to eat when you don't should eat. It's as simple as that.

Activate your creative mind again. Now imagine that you are standing in a beautiful field with tall grass, blowing in your wind. Now imagine that there's a path in front of you, and that path is made up of smooth stones. As you walk along this path, see yourself coming towards a magnificent Japanese temple that was built hundreds of years ago.

The building is well maintained with a fresh coat made of red paint as well as gold trim surrounding the windows and doors. Now make your way up to the front door and feel like the iron handle in your hand on this door is massive as you open it.

So, as you step inside the temple, feel the cool air around you. Also, imagine that the interior of this structure is a work of art, crafted by sheer genius. Now notice that there is a large golden bowl in the center of the room that is set atop a marble column. Now, as you move away from this bowl, it will appear to be illuminated with a ray of sunlight, which is casting down through the window on the rooftop.

As you see, the, reflecting the light like a diamond. Now, you easily remove the gastric band and place it inside the sacred water. So, you can see that it is your favorite color, yet it's a bit worn and tired from all the work that it did for your health. Now imagine the ray of light beaming down and see it begin to dissolve the gastric band until the water is pure. Start to feel lighter than ever, and your stomach smaller, along with your figure, shrinking every day.

Feel the sensations of touch at your fingertips. Move your focus to your abdomen and to all your vital organs. Notice how your belly feels and how it is digesting. Notice your pelvis and hips and the sensations of your weight as it's pressing it down. This should take you into a deeper state of relaxation. Your awareness should go down on each leg, over your knees, move down all the way to your feet, and touch each toe.

CHAPTER 16:

Virtual Gastric Band Sample

Start breathing slowly and deeply.

-

you are lying down, and you are entirely receptive to me

-

You hear my voice mix with your inner voice.

-

My voice is now your voice.

-

Breathe in through your nose and out through your mouth.

Let it create circular and continuous breathing.

-

Feel the air flowing in, filling the lower lungs.

The abdomen swells to the maximum inhalation, so hold your breath for three seconds. Then mentally count to five when you exhale.

-

Follow me:

Inhale deeply 1,2,3.

Exhale slowly: 1, 2, 3, 4, 5.

-

Inhale 1,2,3.

exhale: 1, 2, 3, 4, 5.

-

Every time you exhale, you feel more and more relaxed.

-

Inhale 1,2,3.

exhale: 1, 2, 3, 4, 5.

-

Every time you exhale, you feel more and more relaxed.

-

It will help you think much more clearly by increasing the level of oxygen reaching your brain.

-

you are perfectly calm and relaxed

-

As you continue to breathe and relax, you know your feet and calves' muscles are becoming heavy and comfortable. Let go of the tension and stiffness.

And this pleasant feeling of relaxation begins to spread to your leg muscles. You can go deeper and deeper.

-

I am feeling peaceful and calm.

-

You are perfectly calm and relaxed.

-

You can go deeper and deeper.

-

Feel the sensation in your feet

-

feel the force of gravity pushing them down.

let them go.

-

They are heavily relaxed.

-

Your calves are also massive.

The force of gravity brings them down.

And you also begin to feel heavy and motionless legs.

Perfectly relaxed

you are calm and relaxed.

.

This feeling of relaxation diffuses in the body

-

And every muscle in the abdomen and chest becomes calm and relaxed, free from tension and rigidity.

-

This sensation spreads to the muscles of the back, and the muscles become relaxed and relaxed.

-

Along the spine, the muscles become relaxed and relaxed. One by one. Like a mental massage from the base of the spine to the neck.

-

With every word I say, you feel more relaxed.

-

Go deeper and deeper

-

Enjoy this unique moment where you get inside yourself and get stronger and stronger.

-

This feeling of relaxation spreads to the shoulders and arms.

your right arm is heavy

-

Now your left arm is also massive.

-

Let go of any stiffness, and you may notice a tingling sensation on your fingertips as your arms relax.

-

You feel heavy and relaxed

-

You keep going deeper and deeper

-

Now let go of your thoughts and feel your neck muscles relax entirely, all the way to your head.

-

You're calm and safe, at peace with yourself.

And the tension in your forehead simply begins to melt away.

-

The muscles of the eyebrows are relaxed and relaxed

-

More and more deeply

In a few moments, I'll count from 1 to 3.

When I get to 3, your mind will be ten times calmer and more relaxed

-

Let's start: 1...2...3...

-

A positive feeling spread in you

-

Today will be a special day for you.

The day of the intervention has finally arrived.

-

You find yourself lying on a trolley in a

white surgery room

-

you know you are going to

be changed and that when you wake up you

will be different

-

you will be starting a new life

-

you see figures in green around

you

-

They are slowly moving

-

they are relaxed and perfectly know what they are doing.

Today they will help you change your life.

They are talking to you, asking you to relax, and gently placing a mask on your face

-

you almost feel a hand on your wrist briefly

and you're vaguely aware of the

noises around you and the ceiling lights

-

you're happy at this moment and

somehow you sense something happening on

your tummy

-

you feel something gently spread across

your skin

A slight sensation of pressure and you

can sense that

something is happening inside you.

-

You are inside you and see a white rubber band tie around your stomach, which is now as small as a golf ball.

-

it has all plan with the

greatest of care you feel it is

tested and checked

-

and there's a feeling

of satisfaction in the air

-

it's all over

-

the band fits now, and you can visualize

that band pinched around the entrance

of the stomach

-

That band means a lot to you.

-

You feel safe and secure now.

-

You already feel a sense of contentment and satiety.

-

your new life has just begun

-

You are in front of the mirror.

-

You can see and feel that something is profoundly different.

-

you can feel something different in

your stomach,

there's a tightness there

-

Remember how you used to feel

when did you know you had overeating?

-

remember how it used to have that feel,

and from now on, the smallest bit of food

feels huge

-

your stomach feels full all the time

-

Your life is so good because you've lost weight, and you start to notice how fit and healthy you feel.

-

You took control of yourself, and you are enjoying life.

-

You like to feel healthy and fit

-

Because your stomach is as small as a golf ball now. One bite and you feel full.

-

It's a part of you now.

-

You're in control of your eating habits.

-

The surgery was perfect, and you can finally feel proud of the change.

-

You're delighted with being healthy and fit.

-

Your quality of life has improved.

-

You have much more energy and enthusiasm.

-

You have much more control than many other aspects of your life...

-

Your self-esteem has become much more substantial.

-

With this image of you, you feel more attractive and pleasantly regarded.

-

You keep feeding yourself healthy

-

It is your new image

-

You feel and see your body clearly

You radiate confidence, and you're proud of yourself.

-

You did it; you achieved your goal. It is already a reality

-

I'll count again from 1 to 3. When I get to number 3, you will relax ten times more profoundly, focused, and determined to maintain your new food balance.

Let's start: 1...2...3...

-

You are ten times more focused

-

Your mind is receptive and calm

You feel a positive feeling spreading through your body.

-

You feel more determined than ever before.

-

Repeat after me: My stomach is the size of a golf ball.

-

Repeat after me: I eat the right amount of healthy, nutritious food.

-

Repeat after me: I like the taste of fresh, clear water.

-

Repeat after me: I exercise and stay fit

-

Repeat after me: I eat fruit and vegetables with pleasure.

-

Repeat after me: I feel full after a light, healthy meal.

.

These feelings take root sincerely in your mind and are your reality.

-

Your unconscious mind continues to see this positive outcome

-

You respond much better to lives' difficulties.

And you continue to feel more determined

-

Breathe deeply and slowly.

-

You are living with renewed confidence and courage. Your self-esteem grows more and more.

-

You are satisfied with your gastric band.

It doesn't take much to make you feel full.

-

You think more clearly and remain calm even in the most challenging situations, calmly developing greater inner strength.

-

You can concentrate your mind with confidence and get what you want.

-

In a few moments, I'll count from one to ten. With each number, you'll get more and more awake.

-

At number 8, you'll open your eyes, and at number 10, you'll be awake.

-

1.. 2.. 3.. Wake up.

-

4...5... - wake up...

-

6..7...8 open your eyes....

-

9 – 10

Now you're awake, and your diet is healthy and balanced and you can feel that band around your stomach.

CHAPTER 17:

Self-Hypnosis Techniques to Help You Stay on Track at Home

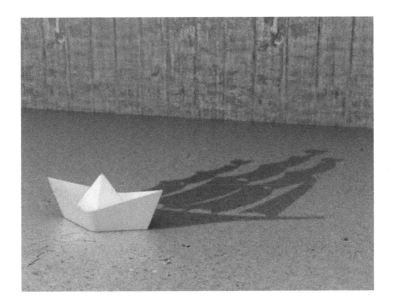

The only significant difference between hypnosis and self-hypnosis is that in the first one, the operator and the subject are two different people. In self-hypnosis, the operator and the issue coincide in the same person.

It is also a fact that learning is more comfortable and faster when done with another person.

The number of times it is necessary to reinforce the procedure depends entirely on you. If you practice the daily self-hypnosis exercise, one or two reinforcement sessions will be sufficient.

But what about those who have no one with whom to share the learning experience of self-hypnosis? What can they do? How can they learn?

Leave your worries aside.

It is possible to use self-hypnosis to solve virtually any type of problem and broaden your consciousness and connect with your innate superior intelligence and creative ability. By using self-hypnosis for the latter purpose, hypnosis can transform into meditation.

Self-hypnosis can also be used in those moments when you feel the need for a higher power to intervene in some situations; then it becomes a prayer. The subtle differences between these forms of self-hypnosis lie in the way thoughts are guided once the state of consciousness itself has altered, that is when the alpha state has reached.

Then I will tell you a fun experience that happened to me with self-hypnosis. I had an appointment with the dentist to have two molars removed. Last night I had conditioned myself to stop the flow of blood.

On the day of the appointment, when sitting in the dentist's chair, I self-reported. When the dentist removed the teeth, I blocked the flow of blood so that it did not flow through the open wound. The dentist was perplexed and kept telling his assistant: «It doesn't bleed.

How is it possible? I don't understand it. I smiled since I couldn't physically smile because of all the devices, cotton, and objects that held my mouth. Besides, I visualized quick and complete healing. After seventy-two hours the swelling had subsided, and the wounds had healed completely;

And now, I will tell you another funny experience that one of my patients had with self-hypnosis.

He was part of a group that participated in an investigation about dreams at the local hospital. Once a week, my patient slept in the hospital with an electroencephalogram (EEG) connected to his head. This was intended to record the waves of their brain activity.

By observing the graph, doctors could establish if they were an alpha, beta, tit, or delta, and they could also state when the patient was sleeping and when he was awake. My client immediately hypnotized himself as soon as he connected to the EEG.

The apparatus recorded a deep alpha state, indicative that the subject was sleeping, although he was fully awake. One of the doctors asked: "What's going on here?" Then the man alternately returned to the beta state, then to alpha, then again to beta, and finally to alpha while the machine registered it.

The changes confused the doctors until the subject told them what he was doing. The response of the doctors cannot reproduce here.

I have devised and written practically all the contents of this guidebook in an alpha state. What does this mean? It means that it is possible to develop an activity and keep your eyes open even if one is in an altered state of consciousness. Think about it for a moment.

It transports us to another state while we are comfortably and quietly sitting with our eyes closed, thinking about a specific objective. But using self-hypnosis in this sense is not easy to achieve since it requires a prolonged period of preconditioning in a hypnotic or auto hypnotic state. Such preconditioning is similar to that used for diet control, but the indications are different; It will be necessary to devise the techniques and suggestions for this case.

And it also requires practice, a lot of practice. Do not forget my words; time and effort will reward with the results. Develop your discipline and stick to it; The results will be a real success.

Guided Daily Meditation in Performing Self-Hypnosis

The experience of this guided meditation will be enhanced if you find yourself in a comfortable and ventilated spot.

Ensure that there is no disturbance from anything or anyone for thirty minutes.

At this particular moment, there is nothing that you need to worry about. You are at peace, and you are safe. You will allow the tensions of the day to dissipate so that you can connect with your inner self. With your eyes closes, breathe deeply and slowly through your nose and then exhale through your mouth. When you breathe in, you are taking all that is good and positive about this world into your body, and when you breathe, you are letting go of all tensions and unnecessary fears.

Now, inhale again. Breathe in slowly through your nose to the count of four.

One, two, three, and four.

With your lungs now full of oxygen, hold your breath for two seconds.

One and two.

And now exhale slowly through your mouth. You need to emit to the count of four.

One, two, three, and four.

When you breathe in, you can slowly feel your diaphragm expand when you feel the air enter your lungs. Breathe in until you feel like your lungs are full of air.

Strive to control the exhalation of air and make sure that you breathe out steadily

You need to continue this cycle of rhythmic breathing.

Inhale to the count for four.

Hold your breath for a count of two.

Exhale your breath to the count of four.

You can resume breathing normally, and you will feel all the tension in your body slowly dissipate.

Acknowledge that your body is now starting to feel more relaxed. Your arms and legs will begin to feel heavier.

Relax the tension in your lower back, middle-back, and your upper back. We often tend to store stress in our shoulders. Learn to release it. When you let go of the tension you feel in your body, you can contact your body relax.

Elongate your neck so that there is a space between your ears and shoulders. When you slowly elongate your neck, you can feel the mattress you are lying on or the chair that you are sitting on support your back.

Now, scan your body and check if there are any areas of tension left. If you feel that there are some, then you need to tighten the muscles in those areas and let go deliberately. Once you do this, you can contact your body to relax. You can feel the tension leaving your body.

Now, you need to go into a state of deep meditation.

To do this, you need to continue the rhythmic breathing exercise.

Imagine that you are now standing in a beautiful meadow with soft rays of sunlight falling on you.

You can see an arched doorway carved into a rising cliff.

Your surroundings look quite peaceful, and you feel good.

You can see golden sandy beaches behind you and azure blue skies above you.

Now, you are slowly making your way to the arched doorway. The door is within your reach; the wood feels warm under your fingers. As you trail your fingers across the door, you can feel a sense of excitement and wonder as you imagine what lies behind the door.

To enter, you need to keep your mind open to the wonders that lie ahead. Reach out and slowly turn the handle of the door.

As you emerge, you can see a lush and beautiful, bright-green rainforest.

A few moments ago, the air felt fresh and pleasant under the canopy and the welcome change from the sun-drenched beach.

Take a deep breath and then exhale to embrace this sense of peace.

As you start to walk forward, you notice a trail that leads through this beautiful rainforest.

As you look up, you can see glimpses of a beautiful blue sky speckled with soft, cotton-like clouds.

Continue scanning the sky all around you.

You are surrounded by majestic mahogany trees that reach up tall towards the zenith.

You marvel at the dark brown bark of the trees that seems to have a pleasantly sweet odor.

Space is limited here, but you are grateful for the narrow trail that leads you through this place of natural wonder.

You can listen to the melodious chirping of birds all around you.

It feels like the forest has come alive around you.

All of these appeals to your senses, and you can experience nature in its pristine form.

Consider if you strip back your own life and where to live more naturally, how much better you will feel.

Only a small percent of sunlight can penetrate onto the floor of this rainforest. So, you move further out in the wilderness; you can see the flashes of exotic blue butterflies dancing around you.

You can hear the melodic sound of running water in the distance and feel compelled to move towards it.

As you take in the wonder of the beautiful nature all around you, you move towards the more massive expanse of the forest area that leads to a delicate stream of water.

There are natural stepping-stones that lead you to a pool of water that looks crystal clear. Green plants surround the pool of water.

You walk closer to the pool, and you notice plants with colorful berries all around.

There are several fruit-bearing plants, and everything looks rich, exotic, and tempting.

You take a bite of these delicious berries, and you can feel a burst of flavors.

Start to concentrate on your breathing. Inhale as you open up your chest and exhale slowly.

It is time that you start to feel good about the person you are. It is time to feel content and embrace pure inner peace. Here in this rainforest, you are free to explore and be the person that you want to be.

Let go of any unhealthy eating habits; it is time to be kind to your body and to nurture and protect your body.

Repeat these affirmations to yourself and believe in each word.

Believe in the message and the power these words have to change your life.

I will change my perception of my body.

I recognize my self-worth.

I will change my eating habits so that I see my food as fuel and nutrients rather than comfort food.

I will exchange binge eating for breathing techniques and guided visualization.

I will start exercising and changing how I look and feel.

I will create an activity diary and plan on how to embrace exercise.

I am ready to face my inner fears and make the necessary positive changes.

Sit quietly for a moment and let these affirmations become a part of you.

It is time to feel positive about your life.

It is time to face any weight issues head-on.

You have the power to do so.

At any time, you can return to this rainforest and experience the wonders of nature. You can find your inner strength and inspiration in this haven.

You are centered, and you retain the feeling of peace and wonder.

Enjoy the moment and the feeling of harmony that you experience.

Breathe in and then out.

Retain your sense of peace and your desire to nurture your body.

Breathe in and out.

You will change your association with food.

Breathe in and out.

Slowly open your eyes on the count of three.

One, two, and three.

Now, you are back in your reality.

Stretch your body slowly and continue to take deep breaths.

Realize how good you feel in this moment.

Remember your desire to improve your fitness and your wellbeing.

Return to this haven of yours whenever you want to improve your health.

GASTRIC BAND HYPNOSIS EXTREME WEIGHT LOSS

CHAPTER 18:

Why Is It Hard to Lose Weight?

For anyone who has ever struggled with weight, life can seem like an uphill battle. It can be downright devastating to see how difficult it can be to turn things around and shed some weight.

The fact of the matter is that losing weight doesn't have to be an uphill battle. Most of this requires you to understand better why this struggle happens and what you can do to help give yourself a fighting chance.

Physiological factors are affecting your ability to lose weight. There are also psychological, emotional, and even spiritual causes that affect your overall body's ability to help you lose weight and reach your ideal weight levels.

The Obvious Culprits

The obvious culprits that are holding you back are diet, a lack of exercise, and a combination of both.

First off, your diet plays a crucial role in your overall health and wellbeing. When it comes to weight management, your diet has everything to do with your ability to stay in shape and ward of unwanted weight.

When it comes to diet, we are not talking about keto, vegan, or Atkins; we are talking about the common foods which you consume and the amounts that you have of each one, which is why diet is one of the obvious culprits. If you have a diet that is high in fat, high in sodium,

GASTRIC BAND HYPNOSIS EXTREME WEIGHT LOSS

and high in sugar, you can rest assured that your body will end up gaining weight at a rapid rate.

When you consume high amounts of sugar, carbs, and fats, your body transforms them into glucose, which storing it in the body as fat. Of course, a proportion of the glucose produced by your body is used up as energy. However, if you consume far more than you need, your body isn't going to get rid of it; your body is going to hold on to it and make sure that it is stored for a rainy day.

Here is another vital aspect to consider: sweet and salty foods, the kind that we love so dearly, trigger "happy hormones" in the brain, namely dopamine. Dopamine is a hormone that is released by the body when it "feels good". And the food is one of the best ways to trigger it, which is why you somehow feel better after eating your favorite meals. It also explains the reason why we resort to food when we are not feeling well, which is called "comfort food", and it is one of the most popular coping mechanisms employed by folks around the world.

This rush of dopamine causes a person to become addicted to food. As with any addiction, there comes a time when you need to get more and more of that same substances to meet your body's requirements.

As a result of diet, a lack of regular exercise can do a number on your ability to lose weight and maintain a healthy balance. What regular exercise does is increase your body's overall caloric requirement. As such, your metabolism needs to convert fat at higher rates to keep up with your body's energy demands.

As the body's energetic requirements increase, that is, as your exercise regimen gets more and more intense, you will find that you will need increased amounts of both oxygen and glucose, which is one of the reasons why you feel hungrier when you ramp up your workouts.

However, increased caloric intake isn't just about consuming more and more calories for the sake of consuming more and more calories; you need to consume an equal amount of proteins, carbs, fats, and vitamins too for your body to build the necessary elements that will build muscle, foster movement and provide proper oxygenation in the blood.

Moreover, nutrients are required for the body to recover. One of the byproducts of exercise is called "lactic acid". Lactic acid builds up in the muscles as they get more and more tired. Lactic acid signals the body that it is time to stop working out or risk injury if you continue. Without lactic acid, your body would have no way of knowing when your muscles have overextended their capacity.

After you have completed your workout, the body needs to get rid of the lactic acid buildup. So, if you don't have enough of the right minerals in your body, for example, potassium, your muscles will ache for days until your body is finally able to get rid of the lactic acid buildup. This example goes to show how proper nutrition is needed to help the body get moving and also recover once it is done exercising.

As a result, a lack of exercise reconfigures your body's metabolism to work at a slower pace. What that means is that you need to consume fewer calories to fuel your body's lack of exercise. So, if you end up wasting more than you need, your body will just put it away for a rainy day. Plain and simple.

The Sneaky Culprits

The sneaky culprits are the ones that aren't quite so overt in causing you to gain weight or have trouble shedding pounds. These culprits hide beneath the surface but are very useful when it comes to keeping you overweight. The first culprit we are going to be looking at is called "stress".

Stress is a potent force. From an evolutionary perspective, it exists as a means of fueling the flight-or-fight response. Stress is the human response to danger. When a person senses danger, the body begins to secrete a hormone called "cortisol". When cortisol begins running through the body, it signals the entire system to prep for a potential showdown. Depending on the situation, it might be best to hightail it out and live to fight another day.

In our modern way of life, stress isn't so much a response to life and death situations (though it can certainly be). Instead, it is the response to cases that are deemed as "conflictive" by the mind. This could be a confrontation with a co-worker, bumper to bumper traffic, or any other type of situation in which a person feels vulnerable in some way.

Throughout our lives, we subject to countless interactions in which we must deal with stress. In general terms, the feelings of alertness subside when the perceived threat is gone. However, when a person is exposed to prolonged periods of stress, any number of changes can happen.

One such change is overexposure to cortisol. When there is too much cortisol in the body, the body's overall response is to hoard calories, increase the production of other hormones such as adrenaline and kick up the immune system's function.

This response by the body is akin to the panic response that the body would assume when faced with prolonged periods of hunger or fasting. As a result, the body needs to go into survival mode. Please bear in mind that the body has no clue if it is being chased by a bear, dealing with a natural disaster, or just having a bad day at the office. Regardless of the circumstances, the body is faced with the need to ensure its survival. So, anything that it eats goes straight to fat stores.

Moreover, a person's stressful situation makes them search for comfort and solace. There are various means of achieving this. Food is one of them. So is alcohol consumption. These two types of pleasures lead to significant use of calories. Again, when the body is in high gear, it will store as many calories and keep them in reserve.

This what makes you gain weight when you are stressed out.

Another of the sneaky culprits is sleep deprivation. In short, sleep deprivation is sleeping less than the recommended 8 hours that all adults should sleep. In the case of children, the recommended amount of sleep can be anywhere from 8 to 12 hours, depending on their age.

Granted, some adults can function perfectly well with less than 8 hours' sleep. Some folks can work perfectly well with 6 hours' sleep, while there are folks who are shattered when they don't get eight or even more hours' sleep. This is different for everyone as each individual is different in this regard.

That being said, sleep deprivation can trigger massive amounts of cortisol. This, fueled by ongoing exposure to stress, leads the body to further deepening its panic mode. When this occurs, you can rest assured that striking a healthy balance between emotional wellbeing and physical health can be nearly impossible to achieve.

Now, the best way to overcome sleep deprivation is to get sleep. But that is easier said than done. One of the best ways to get back on track to a certain degree is to get in enough sleep when you can.

The last sneaky culprit on our list is emotional distress. Emotional distress can occur as a result of any number of factors. For example, the loss of a loved one, a stressful move, a divorce, or the loss of a job can all contribute to large amounts of emotional distress. While all of the situations mentioned above begin as a stressful situation, they can fester and lead to severe psychological issues. Over time, these emotional issues can grow into more profound topics such as General Anxiety Disorder or Depression. Studies have shown that prolonged periods of stress can lead to depression and a condition known as Major Depression.

The most common course of treatment for anxiety and depression is the use of an antidepressant. And guess what: one of the side effects associated with antidepressants is weight. The reason for this is that antidepressants tinker with the brain's chemistry in such a way that they alter the brain's processing of chemicals through the suppression of serotonin transport. This causes the brain to readjust its overall chemistry. Thus, you might find the body unable to process food quite the same way. In general, it is common to see folks gain as much as 10 pounds as a result of taking antidepressants.

As you can see, weight gain is not the result of "laziness" or being "undisciplined". Sure, you might have to clean up your diet somewhat and get more exercise. But the causes we have outlined here ought to provide you with enough material to see why there are less obvious causes that are keeping you from achieving your ideal weight. This is why meditation plays such a key role in helping you deal with stress and emotional strife while helping you find a balance between your overall mental and physical wellbeing.

Ultimately, the strategies and techniques that we will further outline here will provide you with the tools that will help you strike that balance and eventually lead you to find the most effective way in which you will deal with the rigors of your day to day life while being able to make the most out of your efforts to lead a healthier life. You have everything you need to do it. So, let's find out how you can achieve this.

CHAPTER 19:

Weight Loss Tips to Practice Every Day

Keeping up a contemporary, quick-paced way of life can leave a brief period to oblige your necessities. You are moving always starting with one thing then onto the next, not focusing on what your psyche or body truly needs. Rehearsing mindfulness can help you to comprehend those necessities.

When eating mindfulness is connected, it can help you recognize your examples and practices while simultaneously standing out to appetite and completion related to body signs.

Originating from the act of pressure decrease dependent on mindfulness, rehearsing mindfulness while eating can help you focus on the present minute instead of proceeding with ongoing and unacceptable propensities.

Individuals that need to be cautious about sustenance and nourishment are asked to:

➢ Explore their inward knowledge about sustenance—different preferences

➢ Choose sustenance that pleases and support their bodies

➢ Accept explicit sustenance inclinations without judgment or self-analysis

➢ Practice familiarity with the indications of their bodies beginning to eat and quit eating.

The Most Effective Method to Start Eating More Intentionally

Stage 1: Eat Before You Shop. We have all been there. You go with a rumbling stomach to the shop. You meander the passageways, and out of the blue, those power bars and microwaveable suppers start to look truly enticing. "When you're excessively ravenous, shopping will, in general, shut us off from our progressively talented goals of eating in a way that searches useful for the body," says Dr. Rossy. So, even if you feel the slightest craving or urge to eat, get a nutritious bite or a light meal before heading out. That way, your food choices will be made intentionally when you shop, as opposed to propelled by craving or an unexpected sugar crash in the blood.

Stage 2: Make Conscious Food Choices. When you truly start considering where your nourishment originates from, you're bound to pick sustenance that is better for you, the earth, and the people occupied with the expanding procedure portrays Meredith Klein, an astute cooking educator, and Pranaful's author. "When you're in the supermarket, focus on the nourishment source," Klein shows. "Hope to check whether it's something that has been created in this country or abroad and endeavors to know about pesticides that may have been exposed to or presented to people who were developing nourishment." If you can, make successive adventures to your neighborhood ranchers advertise, where most sustenance is developed locally, she recommends.

Stage 3: Enjoy the Preparation Process. "When you get ready sustenance, instead of looking at it as an errand or something you need to hustle through, value the process. You can take a great deal of pleasure in food shopping for items that you know will help you feel better and nourish your body.

Stage 4: "Simply eat". This is something we once in a while do, as simple as it sounds, "simply eat." "Individuals regularly eat while doing different things — taking a gander at their telephones, TVs, PCs, and books, and mingling," claims Dr. Rossy. "While cautious eating can happen when you're doing other stuff, endeavor to' simply eat' at whatever point plausible." She includes that centering the nourishment you're eating without preoccupation can make you mindful of flavors you may never have taken note of. Yum!

Stage 5: Down Your Utensils. When you are done eating, immediately put your dishes and utensils away. This is a way of signaling to yourself that you are done eating (it tends to be much a bit tough to accept). "You're getting a charge out of each chomp that way, and you're focused on the nibble that is in your mouth right now as opposed to setting up the following one," Klein says.

Stage 6: Chew, Chew, Chew Your Food. Biting your sustenance is exceptionally fundamental and not only for, you know, not to stun. "When we cautiously eat our sustenance, we help the body digest the nourishment all the more effectively and meet a greater amount of our dietary needs," says Dr. Rossy. Furthermore, no, we won't educate you how often you've eaten your sustenance. However, Dr. Rossy demonstrates biting until the nourishment is very much separated – which will most likely take more than a couple of quick eats.

Stage 7: Check-In with Your Hunger. You frequently miss the sign that your body sends you during supper when you eat thoughtlessly, for example, when supper time turns into your prime time to make up for lost time with Netflix appears or when you have your supper in a rush. At the end of the day, the one that illuminates you when you begin to feel total. Dr. Rossy proposes ending dinner and taking some time with your craving levels to check-in. "Keep eating in case no doubt about it," she proposes. "In case you're not ravenous yet, spare the nourishment for some other time, manure it, or even discard it." Those remains can make the following day an incredible dinner of care.

Last but not least, we get it; life does not always allow sit-down, completely tuned-in mealtimes. So, if you don't have time for all seven steps, attempt to include one or two in each dinner. "If you have only a little window of time, just try to devote yourself to food," suggests Klein. "Set down your phone, get away from the screen, just be there—you can do that regardless of how much time you have."

Tips in Mindful Eating that Transform how you Relate to Food

We lose ourselves in regular daily existence designs each day. Our propensity for vitality pushes and pulls us to and from, and we are left with minimal opportunity to encounter life in a way that, for this very time, we are completely present.

Sometime in the not so distant future, to-day tasks get more from this autopilot state than others. There are a few things we do so regularly in our lives that we become like automatons, doing them all day every day thoughtlessly and commonly. These exercises incorporate strolling, driving, specific sorts of occupation, and eating.

Yet, these exercises additionally loan themselves to the activity of care, because while these examples are speaking to the draw of propensity vitality, they are likewise the perfect thing to snatch on when in any predefined time we need to turn out to be completely present in our life.

Consideration is both the quality and the activity of getting to be completely present at this very time in our life. It's mindfulness that empowers us to break these standard examples and make a move for a progressively alert and present life.

Eating might be more than whatever another movement that fits the activity of cognizance. This because we discover the flavors we experience when we frequently devour fascinating and various, just as the pleasurable demonstration of eating. Thus, it is through the simple exercise of careful gobbling that we can wake up to our life and discover more harmony and joy all the while.

On occasion, we can likewise identify poor practices with nourishment and eating. These poor propensities can cause us a ton of torment, some even respected issue.

The act of eating mindfully can spark a light on our standard eating and sustenance related propensities. What's more, in doing such, we can ease a lot of the agony on our plate identified with the nourishment.

- **Simply eat mindfully.** Take a minute before eating to see the nourishment's smell, visual intrigue, and even surface. Appreciate the various vibes that go with your feast. This concise minute will help open up your cognizance with the goal that you become all the more completely dynamic in the eating demonstration.

- **Take your time**. Remember to lift your hand/fork/spoon and bite the sustenance itself. Give close consideration to each flavor in your mouth and notice how the nourishment you eat feels and scents. Be completely present for the biting go about as your central matter of (light) focus during cautious eating.

- **Recognize thoughts, feelings, and sensations.** When in your general vicinity of awareness, thoughts, feelings, or different sensations emerge, just be aware of them, recognize their reality, and after that, let them go as though they were gliding on a cloud.

CHAPTER 20:

Hypnotic Meditation to Lose Weight

Notes for the speaker are marked in brackets. This text should be read slowly, with plenty of pauses to allow rest and time for the words to sink into the listener, time for them to become sleepy. Significant pauses have been marked within the text.]

Welcome.

This meditation will guide you into a deep state of relaxation. From that place of peace, you will effortlessly absorb positive affirmations that will help you to lose weight with ease.

Repeat this meditation practice regularly. All you have to do is listen — don't worry about making a conscious effort to sit in formal meditation. Don't feel that you need to solve any problems or come to any great realizations while you listen. And don't worry about whether you're 'doing it right'.

By listening, you are doing it right. You are prioritizing your health. You are showing concern for your sense of calm. You are increasing your innate ability to understand the physical needs of your body.

By simply listening, you are sending a message of self-respect to your subconscious; and every time you repeat the meditation, your subconscious receives that message again. Each time, the message becomes stronger.

And this repetition creates neurological pathways in your brain that make it easier and easier for you to access the power of the positive affirmations you'll work with during this meditation.

[Pause]

Now, start by getting comfortable. Towards the end of this practice, you will start to feel blissfully sleepy, and you'll begin to drift into a deep, peaceful sleep. So, make sure that you're lying down somewhere cozy and safe, where you can happily rest.

Ideally, it's the evening, and you're ready to go to bed for the night. You're in bed. You're a comfortable temperature — if you feel too hot or too cold, then make any adjustments you need to make now; perhaps adding or removing layers of clothing or blankets or turning the heating up or down.

Then lie on your back. Allow your feet to drop out to the side; your legs are relaxed. Rest your right hand on your lower abdomen, and your left hand on your chest.

For the next 90 seconds, bring your awareness to your breath. Don't try to control it or change it; just notice the breath.

Notice the length and depth of the breath. The coolness of the air as it enters at the tip of the nose, and the warmer air leaving your body. Notice whether the breath fills your belly, or your ribcage, or stays even higher up in the chest. And notice the quality of the breath — is it easy? Smooth? Raspy? Does it catch or falter?

There is no right or wrong. Notice the natural rhythm of your breath.

Thoughts will come into your mind — that's fine. Allow the thoughts to come. There's no need to judge them. Let them sit in your mind for a moment, and then gently bring the awareness back to the breath.

[90 second pause]

Good. Now, we'll spend some time using the breath to calm the nervous system and move into a state of deeper relaxation. Learning to harness the power of the breath is incredibly valuable, and it can help you to make positive changes in your habitual ways of living. By cultivating awareness of breath and learning how to deepen and direct the breath, you also cultivate awareness of the whole body.

As this awareness develops, your natural intuition becomes stronger. You become more able to recognize the kinds of food that feel good and nourishing and healthy for your body — the food that can support you in living the energetic and active lifestyle that you want. When you can feel food doing wonderful things for your body, you start to crave that food. Without having to force yourself and without feeling as though you're depriving yourself of anything, you'll start to eat more vegetables and fruits, more lean proteins, and more whole grains.

And you become more in tune to feeling the benefits of exercise. When you can feel how a period of exercise has brought you to life — when you can feel how much stronger your heart feels, and how much more free your lungs feel, and how much extra energy and focus you possess as you glide through the day — then you'll want to exercise. Not because you feel like you should. But because it makes you feel good.

So, before we start to work with the breath, here is your first of three affirmations to help you lose weight and improve your health:

I am going to eat more healthy food because I deserve to feel good.

You do deserve to feel good. Repeat this affirmation three times with me. If you feel comfortable doing so, you could speak them out loud. If not, repeat them silently in your mind. Affirmations are just as powerful when you repeat them silently; what's important is that you focus on them fully.

Remember how you were consciously aware of the natural rhythm of your breath a few minutes ago? Bring that same conscious awareness to this affirmation. Now:

I am going to eat more healthy food because I deserve to feel good.

I am going to eat more healthy food because I deserve to feel good.

I am going to eat more healthy food because I deserve to feel good.

[Pause]

Great. Bring the awareness back to the breath. Take a few easy, natural breaths.

Your right hand is still on your lower abdomen; your left hand on your chest.

With the next inhale, start to breathe into the right hand. The right hand rises with the breath as the belly is blown up like a balloon. Fill the abdomen as much as you can, and then when you can't breathe into the belly anymore, start to exhale. Gently allow the belly to fall; the right hand falls with it.

Again, take a deep, full abdominal breath. The right hand rests on the lower abdomen, so it rises as you inhale and falls slowly as you exhale slowly.

Take three more breaths like this.

Into the right hand.

Out of the right hand.

Into the right hand.

Out of the right hand.

Into the right hand.

Out of the right hand.

Well done. Let go of control of the breath — again, take a couple of easy, natural breaths.

[Pause]

And then we'll start to breathe into the left hand.

With the next inhale, start to fill the chest with air. The chest rises as much as possible — all the way up to the collarbone. The left hand rises as the chest rises. The shoulders may move up slightly.

And when you can't inhale any more air into the chest, start to breathe out. Allow the chest to fall; start at the top, so the collarbone falls first, and then the middle of the chest, and then the ribs fall. The left hand falls with the chest.

Really good. And again: another deep, full breath into the chest. The abdomen stays still — it doesn't rise as you breathe into the chest. And exhale slowly.

Take three more breaths like this.

Into the left hand.

Out of the left hand.

Into the left hand.

Out of the left hand.

Into the left hand.

Out of the left hand.

And then let go of control of the breath and take a few easy, undirected breaths.

[Pause]

Now we'll combine the right hand and the left hand to create a full, deep pattern of breath. This breathing technique works with the full motion of the diaphragm — the big muscle behind your ribcage, which helps your body to control and direct the breath.

Breathing like this has an almost instant effect on the nervous system. It signals to the brain that all is well; there's nothing to worry about, and allows the parasympathetic nervous system to lead. This mechanism of the nervous system gives your body a chance to rest and heal; to digest food, and to restore energy.

This kind of deep, diaphragmatic breath also tones the muscles of the abdominal wall and gently massages the internal organs. So not only does it help you relax, but it also helps you to develop muscle strength and internal wellbeing.

When you've got the hang of this breathing technique, you can repeat your second affirmation with each breath. Your second affirmation is:

I am going to move my body in ways that I enjoy because I deserve to feel good.

[Pause]

Let's begin.

First, breathe into the right hand. The belly rises. When the belly can't rise any more, start to breathe into the left hand. Chest rises. All the way to the collarbone.

And then breathe out of the left hand — so the chest begins to fall first. And then breathe out of the right hand, so the belly falls. Allow the body to soften with that wonderful long exhale.

Great. Now, take a second deep, full breath. Inhale into the right hand; and then into the left hand. All the way up to the collarbone.

Exhale out of the left hand; chest falls. And out of the right hand, belly falls. Enjoy that feeling of softening.

Take three more breaths like this.

Into the right hand; left hand.

Out of the left hand; right hand.

Into the right hand; left hand.

Out of the left hand; right hand.

Into the right hand; left hand.

Out of the left hand; right hand.

Perfect. Now you can start to use your second affirmation.

As you inhale, repeat the first part of the affirmation:

I am going to move my body in ways that I enjoy…

And on the exhale, repeat the second part:

because I deserve to feel good.

Breathe slowly and think the words slowly.

When you're ready, let's do it together five times.

Inhale into the right hand, then the left hand, and repeat:

I am going to move my body in ways that I enjoy…

Exhale out of the left hand, then the right hand, and repeat:

because I deserve to feel good.

Inhale: I am going to move my body in ways that I enjoy…

Exhale: because I deserve to feel good.

Inhale: I am going to move my body in ways that I enjoy…

Exhale: because I deserve to feel good.

Inhale: I am going to move my body in ways that I enjoy…

Exhale: because I deserve to feel good.

Inhale: I am going to move my body in ways that I enjoy…

Exhale: because I deserve to feel good.

And relax. Allow the breath to return to a natural rhythm. No effort in the body at all.

[Pause]

Well done. There is no more physical work to do. Your breathing practice has soothed your nervous system. Your body is calming down and finding its rest state. A state of deep relaxation. A state of complete ease.

Take a moment to enjoy this gentle shift from an active body to a restful body.

[Pause]

Notice the mind beginning to rest as the body rests.

You are moving closer to a deep and peaceful sleep. A wonderfully healing rest. As your nervous system relaxes, your body is already beginning to rebuild cells; to restore wellness. The energy that you've used today is being replenished and renewed.

All of this is already happening.

It takes no conscious work. Your body knows how to do this. All you have to do is be. It is effortless.

Your body knows how to carry you into sleep if you release control and allow it to happen.

You don't need to read books or get a nutritionist's advice to become healthier. You have all the knowledge you need within the systems of your body. The key is listening.

CHAPTER 21:

Positive Impacts of Affirmations

You control the fundamental fixings that make self-hypnosis work for you. These are similar fixings that make your experience of achievement for any objective you pick. Let us take a gander at every component and how you may utilize it to perform for you.

Motivation

Motivation is the vitality of your craving, of what you need. Needing is an inclination that you can control. For the greater part of your life, you have chiefly controlled your craving or needing by restricting it or denying it. You might be truly adept at controlling your wants and needing in certain regions and powerless or natural in others. Since this is a "diet" book, you may have just set yourself up to hear that this "diet" will resemble the others that have mentioned to you what you should deny yourself or breaking point. That is, different diets have mentioned to you what not to need, and the accentuation may have been about "not needing" a few nourishments that you have developed to cherish. Welcome to another method of treating yourself; we will urge you to show signs of improvement at "needing." Denial is excluded from Rapid Weight Loss Hypnosis.

Your motivation is a key factor, one of the fundamental fixings. We need you to center your vitality of needing not toward food yet toward the motivation that unmistakably tells your mind-body what you need it to make: flawless weight. We urge you to get great at needing your ideal weight. Here is a model. Let us state that you are in a pool, and out of nowhere, you take in a significant piece of water. At that time, you need just a single thing, a breath of air. It feels decisive, and a breath of air is the main thing on your mind as of now. The needing is so serious and powerful that it dominates every single other idea and urges you to take the necessary steps to get that breath of air. That is the amount we need you to need the weight and self-perception that you want.

Conviction and Believing

Convictions are those musings and thoughts that are valid for you. They don't need to be deductively demonstrated for you to realize that they generally will be valid for you. Insite that, you know about it or not, your activities, both mindful and subconscious, depend on your convictions. Even though your convictions are contemplations and thoughts, they shape your experience by influencing your activities throughout everyday life. If you accept that creatures make great sidekicks, you most likely have a feline or canine or parrot or a ferret or two. If you accept that espresso keeps you alert around evening time, you likely don't drink espresso before hitting the sack. The power of accepting lets you impact your body in manners that may appear to be bewildering. Fake treatment reactions, where people react to an inactive substance as though it were genuine medicine, are regular instances of how convictions are knowledgeable about the body. If an individual truly accepts that he will get well when taking specific medicine, it will happen whether the tablet contains a prescription or is inactive. Similarly, if an individual truly accepts that he can accomplish high evaluations in school, it will occur. If an individual truly accepts that he can achieve his ideal weight, it will occur.

Recollect your pretend games as a kid. Your capacity to imagine is similarly as solid now as when you were exceptionally youthful. It might be somewhat corroded, and you may require a touch of training, yet when you permit yourself to imagine and let yourself have faith in what you are imagining, you will find a powerful apparatus. You will find this is a brilliantly viable approach to convey your goals, those messages of what you need, to the entirety of the phones and tissues and organs of your body, which react by bringing that goal into reality for you. We can't state this enough: musings are things. The musings, the photos, the thoughts you put in your mind become the messages your self-hypnosis passes on to your mind-body, eventually transforming your ideal body into reality and imagining is picking what to accept and getting retained in those thoughts. Similarly, as an amplifying glass can center beams of daylight, you can center your psychological vitality to make your considerations, thoughts, and convictions genuine for your body.

Desire

You may not generally get what you need, yet you do get what you anticipate. Desires contain the vitality of convictions and become the aftereffects of what is accepted. Here is a case of how to "anticipate." When you plunked to peruse this book, you didn't analyze the seat or couch to test its capacity to hold your weight. You just plunked without contemplating it. You didn't need to consider it, because a piece of you is sure, and has such a great amount of confidence in the seat, that you simply "anticipated" it to hold you. That is the way to expect the ideal body weight you want. Remembering this, be mindful of what you state to yourself as well as other people concerning your body weight desires. "I generally put on weight over the special seasons."

Mind-Body in Focus

Every one of the fundamental fixings can create powerful outcomes when centered inside the mind-body. Nonetheless, when these fixings are adjusted appropriately inside the procedure of self-hypnosis, their viability has amplified a hundredfold. Self-hypnosis is a procedure for creating your world. You may think this sounds mystical or unrealistic. However, that is comparative with what you have encountered as yet in your life. These thoughts might be exceptionally new to you. Here is a case of the "relative" idea of new thoughts. Envision that you are given a personal jet that is flawlessly equipped with sumptuous arrangements and a very much prepared team. It is a brilliant blessing, and you get the opportunity to show this designing wonder to certain people who have seen nothing like it.

Your subconscious (mind-body) utilizes the mix of what you need (motivation), what you accept, and what you expect as a plan for activity. The outcomes are accomplished by your mind-body (subconscious) and not by deduction or breaking down. If an individual contact a virus surface that she accepts is hot, she can create a rankle or consume reaction. Then again, an individual contacting an extremely hot surface reasoning that it is cool may not deliver a consume reaction. Individuals who stroll over hot coals while envisioning that they are cool may encounter a warm physical issue (some minor singing on the bottoms of their feet). Yet, their invulnerable framework doesn't react with a consume (rankling, torment, and so on.) Because their minds advise their bodies how to respond. Once more, it is the arrangement of every one of the three of the basic fixings that make this conceivable:

• Wanting to do it

• Believing it conceivable

• Expecting to be fruitful

This is the way to progress. Your body completes your convictions. Your convictions direct your activities, which like this, shape your experience.

Some portray this procedure as creating your prosperity or creating your involvement with life. In our way of life, we see this depicted inside the motivational and positive mental disposition writing. It very well may be seen in numerous zones of mysticism. You can likewise think back to the people of yore and see it depicted in the provisions of the authentic period. An individual a lot smarter than we are stated, "It will be done unto you as per your conviction." In the current period of integrative medication and brain research, we call it self-hypnosis or mind-body medication. There are currently various logical examinations that exhibit astonishing outcomes for torment control, wound mending, physical modification, and a lot of more medical advantages than we recently suspected conceivable.

Picking Your Beliefs

You can pick your convictions. You may decide to accept what you see, in the feeling of "See it to trust it" or "Truth can be stranger than fiction." This is simple to do. You experience something with your faculties, and that is a natural method of picking whether it is reasonable or not. However, you may likewise decide to trust it first and afterward observe it, which may require some training. The vast majority think that it's simpler to let the world mention to them what is valid or what to accept. The TV, media, papers, books, instructors, and specialists besiege us with what to accept. You grew up finding out about the world and yourself from numerous outside sources. This prompted a recognizable example of watching and accepting data about the world from outside yourself, and you picked which data to make a piece of your conviction framework. This included convictions about your body. For instance, when your stomach makes a thundering sound, you accept that it implies you are ravenous. Or then again, you feel queasy and trust you are wiped out. Both of these are instances of watched occasions: you watched an association once and decided to trust it.

In Rapid Weight Loss Hypnosis, we are suggesting that you turn that training around with this thought: "Trust it, and you will see it." This implies you initially pick what to accept, and afterward, your body follows up on it as evidence and makes it genuine, you would say. One of the significant messages we trust you will get from this book is that your mind-body hears all that you hear, all that you state, all that you think, picture, or envision in your mind, and it can't differentiate between what is genuine and what you envision. It follows up on what you need and anticipate. In light of this, which of these announcements would assist you with encountering the ideal weight you want: "I simply take a gander at food and put on weight" or "I can eat anything, and my weight remains the equivalent"? The last mentioned. In any case, which articulation do you by and by accept to be valid for you? Once more, it will be done unto you as indicated by your conviction. We will assist you with the thoughts, language, and pictures that plan compelling hypnotic proposals, yet you have all-out command over what you decide to accept.

As you read the thoughts of this book and hear the hypnotic recommendations offered during the trancework on the sound, you will settle on numerous decisions for yourself. We wholeheartedly urge you to decide to trust it so you will see it for yourself. Your subconscious (mind-body) can't differentiate and will follow up on what you select in any case. Why not select what you truly need?

The Energy of Emotions

Not all considerations and convictions show themselves in your experience. Just those that have the vitality of your sentiments (feelings), alongside your conviction and your desire that something will occur, will show themselves. Your sentiments or feelings are a type of vitality that impacts this procedure of creation.

CHAPTER 22:

Increase Your Wellbeing with 100 Positive Affirmations

1. I am healthy, wealthy, and clever

2. I let go of the illness, I am not ill

3. Thanks to my creator and everyone in my life.

4. I am grateful for all the bounty that I already enjoy

5. Every day I grow energetically and vibrantly

6. I only give my body the necessary nutritious food

7. My body is my temple

8. You can always maintain a healthy weight

9. I deserve to enjoy perfect health

10. Act to be healthy

11. I respect my body and am willing to exercise

12. Affirmation for Rapid and Natural Weight Loss

13. My body is beautiful and healthy

14. I choose healthy and nutritious foods

15. I like to exercise, and I do it frequently

16. Losing weight is easy and even fun

17. I have confidence in myself

18. I am now sure of myself

19. I feel confident to succeed

20. From day to day, I am more and more confident

21. I am sure to reach my goal

22. I want to be a noble example

23. I believe in my value

24. I have the strength to realize my dreams

25. I am really adorable

26. I trust my inner wisdom

27. Everything I do satisfies me deeply

28. I trust the process of life

29. I can free the past and forgive

30. No thought of the past limits me

31. I get ready to change and grow

32. I am safe in the Universe, and life loves me and supports me

33. With joy, I observe how life supports me abundantly and provides me with more goods than I can imagine.

34. Freedom is my divine right

35. I accept myself and create peace in my mind and my heart

36. I am a loved person, and I am safe.

37. Divine Intelligence continually guides me in achieving my goals

38. I feel happy to live

39. I create peace in my mind, and my body reflects it with perfect health

40. All my experiences are opportunities to learn and grow

41. I flow with life easily and effortlessly

42. My ability to create the good in my life is unlimited

43. I deserve to be loved because I exist

44. I am a being worthy of love

45. I dare to try, and I'm proud of it

46. I choose to really love myself

47. I love myself and accept myself completely

48. I am ready to try new things

49. There are things I can already do, I just need to start even though I'm not ready yet

50. I am much more capable than I think

51. As I love myself, I allow others to love me too ...

52. I accumulate more and more confidence in myself

53. I am unique and perfect as I am

54. I am wonderful

55. I'm proud of everything I've accomplished

56. I do not have to be perfect, I just need to be myself

57. I feel able to succeed

58. I give myself permission to go out of my role as a victim and take more responsibility for my life

59. The past is over, I now have control of my life, and I move

60. I am my best friend

61. I am able to say "no" without fear of displeasing

62. I choose to clean myself of my fears and my doubts

63. Fear is a simple emotion that cannot stop me from succeeding

64. Every step forward I make increases my strength

65. My hesitations give way to victory

66. I want to do it, I can do it

67. I am capable of great things

68. There is no one more important than me

69. I may be wrong but that I can handle it

70. With confidence, I can accomplish everything

71. I allow myself to have a lot of fun

72. I deserve to be seen, heard, and shine

73. I deserve love and respect

74. I choose to believe in myself

75. I allow myself to feel good about myself and trust myself

76. I reduce measures quickly and easily

77. I can maintain my ideal weight without many problems

78. My body feels light and in perfect health

79. I'm motivated to lose weight and stay

80. Every day I reduce measures and lose weight

81. I fulfill my weight loss goals

82. I lose weight every day, and I recover my perfect figure

83. I eat like a thin person

84. I treat my body with love and give it healthy food

85. I choose to feel good inside and out

86. I feed myself only until I am satisfied, I don't saturate my food body

87. I know how to choose my food in a balanced way.

88. I feed slowly and enjoy every bite.

89. I am the only one who can choose how I eat and how I want to see myself.

90. It is easy for me to control the amount of what I eat.

91. I learn to have habits that lead me to my ideal weight.

92. Being at my ideal weight makes me feel healthy and young.

93. My body is very grateful and quickly reflects all the care I have with him.

94. My body reflects my perfect health.

95. I feel better every day

96. Being at my ideal weight motivates me to do other things that I like.

97. The human body is moldable, and I am the artist of my body.

98. Every day I eat with awareness.

99. I consume the calories needed to have an ideal weight and a healthy body.

100.   Every day I like the way I feel.

CHAPTER 23:

Deep Sleep for Weight Loss

There are several things you know you should follow when you are aiming to lose that extra weight. You eliminate junk foods and sugar from your diet and include lots of complex carbohydrates, lean proteins, and vegetables. You try to exercise as much as you can throughout the day and go to the gym regularly. However, what you don't realize is that one of the essential parts of losing weight is getting adequate sleep.

The Daily Express had reported that good sleep is the best recipe to reduce weight. It also said that people who can decrease their stress levels and get about 8 hours of sleep every night could double their weight loss. It's true: getting enough sleep can help you lose weight.

How Does Sleep Benefit Weight Loss?

The amount of sleep you can get becomes as essential as exercise and diet when you are trying to lose weight. Here are some reasons why sleeping properly can help you in losing weight:

· Inadequate amount of sleep tends to increase your appetite – Several studies have shown that people who get an inadequate amount of sleep have an increased appetite. This might be caused by the impact of sleep on the hormone leptin and ghrelin. These are 2 of the essential hunger hormones present in the human body. The hormone ghrelin, which is released in your stomach, signals to your brain that you're hungry. When your stomach is empty before you start eating, the level of ghrelin increases, while it decreases after you consume. The other hunger hormone leptin is released from fat cells. This hormone signals fullness to your brain and suppresses your hunger. In the absence of adequate sleep, your body reduces the production of leptin while increasing the ghrelin production, thus increasing your appetite and making you hungry.

· Inadequate sleep is a significant risk factor for obesity and weight gain – Shortage of sleep has been linked with weight gain and a higher BMI. Studies have shown that although people have different sleep requirements when they get less than 7 hours of sleep every night, it can cause weight changes. Moreover, several sleep disorders, such as sleep apnea, get worse due to weight gain. Therefore, a shortage of sleep can result in weight gain, which worsens sleep quality.

· Sleep helps prevent resistance to insulin – Your cells can become resistant to insulin because of poor sleep. The hormone insulin transports sugar from your blood into your body's cells so that your body can use it in the form of energy. However, if your cells become resistant to insulin, the sugar fails to enter the cells and remains in your bloodstream. To compensate for this, more insulin is produced by your body, which ends up making you feel hungrier. As a result, your body stores the extra calories as fat. Resistance to insulin can cause both weight gain and type-2 diabetes.

· Sleep helps you make healthy choices by fighting cravings – Sleep deprivation can change the way your brain works,

making it more difficult for you to resist cravings and make healthy choices. Lack of sleep dulls the activity of your brain's frontal lobe, which makes decisions and controls impulses. Moreover, when you're sleep-deprived, the reward centers of your brain get more stimulated by food. Studies also suggest that inadequate sleep can increase your affinity for high-calorie foods.

· Inadequate sleep can reduce your resting metabolism – The number of calories burnt by your body when you are at rest is known as your resting metabolic rate or RMR. Studies reveal that lack of sleep can decrease your RMR. In one study where fifteen men were kept awake for twenty-four hours, their resting metabolic rate found to be five percent less than usual, and their metabolic rate was after consuming food was found to be twenty percent lower. Moreover, lack of sleep can also result in muscle loss.

· Sleep can increase physical activity – Poor sleep can result in daytime fatigue, which can decrease your motivation to exercise. Moreover, it's more likely that you will get tired quickly while applying. A study done on fifteen people revealed that when the participants were deprived of sleep, the intensity and amount of their physical exercise reduced. Thus, getting an adequate amount of proper sleep can help improve your athletic performance.

Therefore, to maintain your weight, you must get quality sleep along with the right diet and exercise. The way your body responds to food can dramatically be altered by inadequate sleep. For starters, as your appetite grows, it will become difficult for you to resist temptations and control your portion size. This turns into a vicious cycle. A shortage of sleep will make you gain weight, and it will make it harder for you to get adequate sleep. However, following healthy sleeping habits can help you lose weight and maintain a healthy body.

CHAPTER 24:

Gastric Band Hypnosis for Food Addiction

O besity is a growing epidemic in the world today. It is prevalent among adults, but the rate of increase in obesity among children is profoundly worrying. Obesity has contributed to the increased use of aids, which can support weight loss boosters like metabolism. Food is the survival function of any human being. But maybe there are one or more things like candy or chocolates that you like more than two or three times a day. You may not know, but these may be indicators of addiction to food. You may also be addicted to fast food if you have more fast food than usual.

Today's food addiction is like an epidemic. The biggest concern is that many people don't even know that they have a disease and are still over-alimenting. The effect is that a person is addicted to food and consumes a significant number of calories. The explanation that most overweight food consumers do not lose weight is due to their eating habits.

Physicians identify these addicts as people with binge eating disorders. It can lead to severe problems such as diabetes, heart disorders, kidney disorders, and even depression. Food addiction's key symptoms include a constant sense of hunger, shifting in mood, and fluctuation in weight.

Therapy and therapy are the only way to handle the issue of food addiction. You should find a doctor that can help you lose weight in a clinic. If you see a therapist, you can know that you are not the only one with this dilemma that can alleviate the shame. A therapist will help you find out why you are addicted and help you to conquer it with simple methods. He will also teach you how to lose weight healthily.

One must also recognize that it is a long-term process. Hence, patience is essential when you meet with a therapist and a psychologist and must obey their advice appropriately and promptly. Some organizations run rehabilitation services for eating disorders. You can join any of these groups as well. You need to get out of your comfort zone to help yourself deal with the addiction and control your appetite to get rid of unhealthy foods from your diet.

What Foods Are Most Likely to Be Addictive?

The response is frustrating: typically, the most delicious. A researcher involved in food dependency takes stock of the problem in a recent report. His findings suggest that refined, fat, and high glycemic foods are "more commonly correlated with food abuse behavior." Here are several examples:

· Pizza: Pizza is close at the top of the list with its delicious mix of carbs, salt, and fat. "How many spikes ought I to eat?" you ever wondered. The answer: at most, but how to avoid the pizza call. It typically contains more fat per bite than other healthier foods, consisting of many refined ingredients. If you combine all this with salt, you will get a great recipe to get dopamine straight to the next tip. You know it's not essential, but then your brain tells you.

· Treats: Sugar and fat will quickly induce the brain to desire more, candy, cookies, cake, and ice cream. A salty meal is a common practice with a sweet dessert, but it is not a safe option. It allows you to consume sugar and consume more than you need if your food option is unhealthy. Therefore, you can have the extra benefit of calories, fat, and sugar.

· Fried foods: this example is not surprising considering what we already know. Freezes and potato chips are salted and usually fried in oils that do not do your body or brain a lot of good. Although some fried foods are delicious, they are unhealthy and vulnerable to food addiction.

What About Carbonated Drinks?

Soft drinks and fatty and salty foods can be addictive. Research carried out in 2007 found a secure connection between the use of carbonated foods and increased energy intake, that is, the consumption of more calories a day, the existing association between them, and the adverse effects on diet and health well as weight gain. Carbonated beverages were often associated with a decreased consumption of calcium and other nutrients. Consumers of soft drinks are even more at risk for long-term medical issues.

How do carbonated drinks become so addictive? The mystery is straightforward to unwrap: regular carbonated drinks are filled with sugar and often also with caffeine.

Studies show that such beverages can help with weight gain because artificial sweeteners are designed to cause similar reactions in the brain. One research explicitly indicates that individuals who consume artificial sweeteners may have an increased desire for sugar, choose sugar over healthier foods, and be less motivated by health.

Steps to Control Food Addiction

1. Identify the Foods You Are Addicted To

The most addictive foods are rich in sugars, fat, flour, and sodium. Not to mention caffeinated foods such as coffee, soft drinks, and chocolate.

2. Make a Healthy Replacement

When the urge to satisfy your addiction hits, eat another healthier food. When sugar levels drop, hunger hits, instead of consuming sugar, eat healthy protein every 3 or 4 hours, such as cashew or Pará nuts. Eliminate soft drinks (even dietary ones) and industrialized juices (which have a high sugar). Take unsweetened water and natural juices instead.

Some liquids, like orange juice, are very caloric. Prefer to eat the fruit with bagasse.

Don't forget breakfast. It is the most important meal of the day. It must contain fruits, cereals, and protein. When we do not eat breakfast, the desire to eat the food we are addicted to can be uncontrollable.

3. Drink, Instead of Eating

A glass of water may be the solution to what you think is hunger, but which is thirst.

4. Occupy Your Time and Your Mind

Avoid doing nothing when you are not working or studying. The more things you have to do, the less time you'll have to think about food.

5. Practice Physical Exercises

Eating something we like a lot produces a sense of pleasure. Physical activities also provoke such feelings. The difference is that after physical activity, you will feel satisfied and in a good mood, while you will feel sad and guilty when you overeat. Exercising boosts self-esteem and overeating ultimately affects self-esteem.

6. Buy Healthy Foods

When shopping at the supermarket, avoid going through the candy aisles, especially if your object of destruction is in that aisle. Make a list of suitable products for your health and follow them when shopping.

7. Learn or Relearn How to Chew

Chew slowly and thoroughly. Proper chewing produces satiety and good digestion. The stomach sends a satiety message to the brain after 20 minutes from the start of the meal. The more you chew, the longer it will take to eat. You will be sated with a lot less than you think. Therefore, you must allow about 30 minutes to eat your main meals.

8. Seek Expert Advice

Binge eating is a disease, so it needs to be adequately treated. Without the support of a psychologist, nutritionist, and other specialists, you will find it challenging to carry out the treatment until the end. Relapses can be successive, which can be a reason for discouragement and withdrawal.

Overcome Your Food Addiction and Lose Weight!

When you hear the word "addiction," you mostly think of opioids or smoking addiction. They stop little and think about becoming food addicted. You can get addicted as quickly as you can with medicines. Depression plays a significant part, but there are many explanations about why it is possible. Some of the reasons are that you are bored and want to have some food or mental issues you don't know. What would you do if you know you are food-suffering now?

You must first take a deep breath and know it's okay. Don't let panic and anxiety stop you from doing the right thing in your path. Breathe out now. You may want to do it for a couple of seconds before you feel relaxed. You have to focus on thinking before you plan to do something and realize that you can conquer this addiction. The moment you continue to live negatively with food is when you are addicted. Know, "I lose weight, and I'm safe." Don't think about saying, "I should lose weight," even if it's in the present and "now" tense, making it past tense. Now that you are right, the next move should not be such a challenge.

Find a doctor who can help you succeed in a weight loss plan. Joining a program helps you because you're conscious that you're not alone, and you can find out several times what made you addicted to food in the first place. You will be taught a healthier way to lose weight and conquer your addiction by going to a clinic. At first, it might not be convenient, but finally, it is very rewarding.

You should throw out all your fast food while you're doing the plan. This will be a significant change for many. Throwing out the wrong food will build an even better attitude because you know that you can do it for real.

How to Overcome Junk Food Cravings with Weight Loss Hypnosis

1. "Reset" Your Fast Food Attachment

Weight loss hypnotherapy is one of the easiest ways to improve your mindset towards unhealthy food without experiencing excessive cravings or feelings of inadequacy.

For most people, consuming fast food is either an impulsive option or an emotional one. They need to exercise will to stop the momentum, and this process will typically lead to a feeling that they robbed or limited.

You will alter the response mechanism through hypnosis. Ethical behaviors are fun, and the practice improves. You learn to cope well, which means you don't have to rely on food for comfort. Resetting the connection frees your mind and body so that you have fun during weight loss.

2. Get Motivated

The right inspiration will assist you in moving mountains. You have to have the right reasons if you want to get rid of fast food forever.

Most people don't realize that eating nutritious foods benefits their physical wellbeing even more than appearance. By hypnosis of weight loss, people know what the right encouragement is and what important role it plays in the process of weight loss.

Success implies constructive encouragement. You need not confine yourself to discovering the world of balanced eating. You will find it incredibly non-traumatic and even enjoyable if you are enthusiastic about the transition.

3. Get in Touch with Your Emotions

the time or find it challenging to deal with stress in any other way. Contacting inner feelings and unresolved problems will have the power and motivation never to feel the need for fast food.

Have you deemed a compulsive overeater? Were you seen as a fast-food by others? If so, you still have emotional baggage to deal with.

CHAPTER 25:

Eat Healthy and Sleep Better with Hypnosis

Make yourself comfortable.

Find the perfect sleep position.

Inhale through your nose and exhale through your mouth.

Again, inhale through your nose and this time as you exhale, close your eyes.

Repeat this one more time and relax.

Sharpen your breathing focus.

Find stillness in every breath you take, relieve yourself from any tension, and relax.

Let your body relax, soften your heart, quiet your anxious mind, and open to whatever you experience without fighting.

Simply allow your thoughts and experiences to come and go without grasping at them.

Reduce any stress, anxiety, or negative emotions you might have, cool down become deeply and comfortably relaxed.

That's fine.

And as you continue to relax, you can begin the process of reprogramming your mind for your weight loss success because with the right mindset, then you can think positively about what you want to achieve. It begins with changing your mindset and attitude, because the key to losing weight all starts in the mind. One of the very first things you must throw out the window (figuratively) before you start your journey to weight loss is negativity. Negative thinking will just lead you nowhere. It will only pull your moods down, which might trigger emotional eating. Thus, you'll eat more, adding up to that unwanted weight instead of losing it. Remember that you must need to break your old bad habits, and one of them is negative self-talk. You need to change your negative mental views and turn them into positive ones. For example, instead of telling yourself after a few days of workout that nothing is happening or changing, tell yourself that you have done a set of physical activities you have never imagined you can or will do. Make it a point to pat yourself on the back for every little progress you make every day, may it be five additional crunches from what you did yesterday. Understand and accept that this process is a complete transformation, a metamorphosis if you will. This understanding is going to make the process smoother and less painful.

Aside from being positive, you should also be realistic. Don't expect an immediate change in your body. Keep in mind that losing weight is not an overnight thing. It is a long-term process and gradual progress. Set and focus on your goals to keep that negativity at bay.

Don't compare yourself to others, because it will not help you attain your goals in losing weight. First and foremost, keep in mind that each one of us has different body types and compositions. There is a certain diet that may work on you, but not so much for the others. Possibly, some people might need more carbohydrates in their diet, while you might need to drop that and add more protein in your meals. Each one of us is unique. Therefore, your diet plan will surely differ from the person next to you.

Comparing yourself to other people's progress is just a negative thought and will just be unhelpful to you. Remember, always keep a positive outlook and commit to it before you start your diet. For the sake of your long-term success, leave the comparison trap. You're not exactly like the people you idolize, and they're not exactly like you, and that's perfectly fine. Accept that, embrace that and move on with your personal goals.

Be realistic in setting your goals. Think about small and easy to achieve goals that will guide you towards a long term of healthy lifestyle changes. Your goals should be healthy for your body. If you want to truly lose weight and keep it off, it will be a slow uphill battle, with occasional dips and times you'll want to quit. If you expect progress too fast, you will eventually not be able to reach your goals and become discouraged. Don't add extra obstacles for yourself, plan your goals carefully.

If possible, try to find someone who has similar goals as you and work on them together. Two is always better than one and having someone who understands what you are undergoing can be such a relief! An added benefit of having a partner-in-crime (or several) is that you can always hold each other accountable. Accountability is one thing that is easy to start being lax after the first few weeks of a new weight loss program, especially if results aren't quite where you want them to be.

Write down a realistic timetable that you can follow. Start a journal about your daily exercises and meal plan. You can cross out things that you have done already or add new ones along the way. Plot your physical activities. Make time and mark your calendar with daily physical activities. Try to incorporate at least a 15-minute workout on your busy days.

When you become aware of a thought or belief that pins the blame for your extra weight on something outside yourself, if you can find examples of people who've overcome that same cause, realize that it's decision time for you. Choose for yourself whether this is a thought you want to embrace and accept. Does this thought support you living your best life? Does it move you toward your goals, or does it give you an excuse not to go after them?

If you determine your thought no longer serves you, you get to choose another thought instead. Instead of pointing to some external, all-powerful cause for you being overweight, you can choose something different. Track your progress by writing down your step count or workouts daily to keep track of your progress.

Celebrate and embrace your results. Since the path to a healthy lifestyle is mostly hard work and discipline, try to reward yourself for every progress, even if it is small. Treat yourself for a day of pampering, travel to a place you have been wanting to visit, go hiking, have a movie date with friends, or get a new pair of shoes. These kinds of rewards provide you gratification and accomplishments that will make you keep going. Little things do count, and little things also deserve recognition. But keep in mind that your rewards should not compromise your diet plan.

You can also do something like joining an athletic event, a fun run, where you can meet new people that share the same ideals of a healthy lifestyle. You get to learn more about weight loss from others and also share your knowledge. You need to find a source of motivation and keep that source of motivation fresh in your mind, so you don't forget why you embarked on this journey to begin with.

As you focus on your journey of weight loss, keep your stress at bay because too much stress is harmful to the body in many ways, but it also can cause people to gain weight. When the body is under stress, the body will automatically release many hormones and among one of them is cortisol. When the body is under duress and stress, cortisol is released, it can ignite the metabolism for a period of time. However, if the body remains in stressful conditions, the hormone cortisol will continue to be released and actually slow down the metabolism resulting in weight gain.

Everyone experiences stress; there is just no getting around that fact. However, minimizing stressors, as well as learning how to manage the stress in your life will not only help you with losing weight, but it will also make you a more attractive you! High stress in anyone's life often brings out the worst in people. When you are trying to get a man, you want them to see the best of you, not the stressed out you. While you are decreasing your stress level, you will want to increase the amount of sleep you get each night. Lack of sleep is a link to weight gain and because of this, ensuring adequate and appropriate sleep is crucial when trying to lose weight. Sleep is vital for the well-being of the body and the ability for the mind to function, but it is also related to maintaining weight. If you are tired, make sure you sleep, rest or relax, so you are not prone to gaining weight. When a person gets more sleep, the hormone leptin will rise, and when this happens the appetite decreases, which will also decrease body weight.

Gratitude is important in this journey because it teaches you how to make peace with your body, no matter what shape, size or weight it has at the moment. It makes you look at your body with full acceptance and love, saying: "I'm grateful for my body the way it is." It stops you from beating yourself up for being overweight, unhealthy, or out of shape. Be grateful for this learning experience, accept yourself the way you are, and take massive action to get your balance back.

When you express gratitude, you vibrate on a higher energy level, you are positive and happy, and you are simply in a state of satisfaction.

The more things you can find to be grateful for during your weight loss journey, the easier it will be to maintain a positive attitude and keep your motivation up.

It will also get you past those tough moments when you are feeling demotivated to take action and stick to the exercising or eating plan.

This means that you start expressing gratitude for the aspects of your body you would like to have, as if you already have them now. Be grateful for your sexy legs and slim waist. Be grateful for your increased energy levels and strength. Be grateful for the ability to wear smaller clothes. You get the drill. Feel the positive energy of gratitude flowing through your body as you imagine these things are true. By going through this exercise you'll notice the positive change in your thought patterns.

With the level of personal growth you will achieve and the habits you will change in this session of hypnosis, you will feel like a completely different person. You will have more power, self–confidence, and love yourself more than you ever thought possible before. That's a change from the inside out. That's what lasts. And, at the end of the day, that's what truly matters.

Take a deep breath and allow your breath to return its natural rate as you return to your normal consciousness.

As you continue to breathe, note that, right now, at this moment, you have no worries. You are just a relaxed body. Any distractions that arise while you tell yourself this can wait.

Repeat the following phrases:

- I am relaxed

- I am balanced

- I can deal with any worries later

- I am relaxed

- I am balanced

The whole earth supports you in your relaxation and balance. Feel yourself supported and held.

Feel that everything you have done in your life has brought you to this moment without errors or mistakes.

This moment is perfect.

CHAPTER 26:

Deep Relaxing techniques

Since we have seen that emotions are the first obstacle to a healthy and correct relationship with food, we are going to look specifically at the most suitable techniques to appease them. Not only is that, these techniques very important to make hypnosis deeply effective in order to achieve the desired goals.

In fact, autogenic training is one of the techniques of self-hypnosis. What does self-hypnosis mean? As the word suggests, it is a form of self-induced hypnosis. Beyond the various techniques available, all have the objective of concentrating a single thought object. To say it seems easy, but it is incredible how, in reality, our mind is constantly distracted and even overlaps distant thoughts between them. This leads to emotional tension with repercussions in everyday life.

Other self-hypnosis techniques that we will not deal with in-depth include Benson's and Erickson's.

Benson's is inspired by oriental transcendental meditation. It is based on the constant repetition of a concept in order to favor a great concentration. Specifically, he recommends repeating the word that evokes the concept several times. It is the easiest and fastest technique ever. It really takes 10-15 minutes a day. Just because it's so simple doesn't mean it's not effective. And you will also need to familiarize yourself with it. Especially for those who are beginners with self-hypnosis. In fact, this could be the first technique to try right away to approach this type of practice.

You sit with your eyes closed in a quiet room and focus on breathing and relax the muscles. Therefore continually think about the object of meditation. If your thought turns away, bring it back to the object. To be sure to practice this self-hypnosis for at least 10 minutes, just set a timer.

Erickson's is apparently more complex. The first step involves creating a new self-image that you would like to achieve. So we start from something we don't like about ourselves and mentally create the positive image that we would like to create.

In our specific case, we could start from the idea of us being overweight and transform that idea into an image of us in perfect shape, satisfied with ourselves in front of the mirror.

Then we focus on three objects around the subject, then three noises, and finally three sensations. It takes little time to concentrate on these things. Gradually decrease this number. Therefore 2 objects, 2 noises, and 2 sensations. Better if the objects are small and bright and unusual sensations, which are hardly paid attention. For example, the feeling of the shirt that we wear in contact with our skin. You get to one, and then you leave your mind wandering. We take the negative image we have and calmly transform it mentally into the positive one. At the end of this practice, you will feel great energy and motivation.

Autogenic Training

Autogenic training is a highly effective self-induced relaxation technique without external help. It is called "training" because it includes a series of exercises that allow the gradual and passive acquisition of changes in muscle tone, vascular function, cardiac and pulmonary activity, neuro-vegetative balance, and state of consciousness. But don't be frightened by this word. His exercises do not require a particular theoretical preparation nor a radical modification of one's habits. Practicing this activity allows you to live a profound and repeatable experience at all times.

Autogenic means "self-generating," unlike hypnosis and self-hypnosis, which are actively induced by an operator or the person himself.

In essence, the goal is to achieve inner harmony so that we can best face the difficulties of everyday life. It is a complementary tool to hypnosis. The two activities are intertwined. Practicing both of them allows for a better overall experience. In fact, hypnosis helps well to act directly on the subconscious. But in order for hypnosis to be effective, it is necessary to have already prepared an inner calm such that there is no resistance to the instructions given by the hypnotherapist. The origins of autogenic training are rooted in the activity of hypnosis. In the latter, there is an exclusive relationship between hypnotist and hypnotized. Those who are hypnotized must, therefore, be in a state of maximum receptivity in order to be able to reach a state of constructive passivity in order to create the ideal relationship with the hypnotist.

Those who approach autogenic training and have already undergone hypnosis sessions can deduce the main training guidelines from the principles of hypnosis. The difference is that you become your own hypnotist. You must, therefore, assume an attitude of receptive availability towards you. Such activity also allows a higher spiritual introspection, feeling masters of one's emotional state. This undoubtedly brings countless advantages in everyday life.

So I usually suggest everyone try a hypnosis session and then do a few days of autogenic training before they start using hypnosis again on a daily basis. It's the easiest way to approach the relaxation techniques on your own and start to become familiar with the psycho-physical sensations given by these practices. Mine is a spontaneous suggestion. If you have tried meditation and relaxation techniques in the past, you can also go directly into guided hypnosis. In any case, autogenic training can be useful regardless of the level of familiarity with these practices.

It is clear that if you have little time in your days, it makes no sense to put so much meat on the fire. Let's remember that they are still relaxation techniques. If we see them too much as "training," we could associate obligations and bad emotions that go against the principle of maximum relaxation. So I'm not saying do autogenic training and hypnosis every day, 10 push-ups, crunches, and maybe yoga, and then you will be relaxed and at peace with your body. This approach is not good. It is about finding your balance and harmony in a practice that has to be pleasant and deliberate.

Basic Autogenic Training Exercises

The basic exercises of the A.T. are classically divided into 6 exercises, of which 2 fundamental and 4 complementary. Before the 6 exercises, you practice an induction to calm and relaxation, while at the end a recovery and then awakening.

These exercises are considered as consecutive phases to be carried out in each session. It is not mandatory to carry out all the steps together. Especially initially each exercise will have to be understood individually. But if you intend to stop, for example, in the fourth exercise and not do all of them, you will necessarily have to do the other 3 exercises in the same session first. The duration of the session remains unchanged, however, because when you add exercises, you will make each phase last less.

First exercise - "The heaviness." It s a very useful exercise to overcome psychophysical problems related to muscular tensions that derive from emotional tensions.

Second exercise - "The heat." It serves to relieve circulatory problems, in all cases where there is a problem of reduced blood flow to the extremities.

Third exercise - "The heart." It is a highly suggestive exercise that allows you to regain contact with that part of the body that we traditionally deal with emotions.

Fourth exercise - "The breath." It produces a better oxygenation of the blood and organs.

Fifth exercise - The solar plexus. It helps a lot of those who suffer from digestive problems.

Sixth exercise - The Fresh Forehead. Produces a brain constriction vessel that can be very useful to reduce headaches, especially if linked to physical or mental overload.

Recommended Positions

The following positions are suitable for both autogenic training and hypnosis and relaxation techniques in general. I suggest initially to use the lying down position and to use it later in hypnosis for virtual gastric bandaging in order to simulate the position on the surgical couch.

Lie Down

This position, at least at the beginning, is the most used for its comfort. You lie on your back (face up) and your legs slightly apart with your toes out. The arms are slightly detached from the torso and are slightly bent. The fingers are detached from each other and slightly arched.

On the Armchair

You sit with a chair attached to the wall. Your back is firmly against the backrest, and your head rests against the wall. You can place a cushion between your head and the wall.

Alternatively, you can use a high chair to rest your head-on. The feet should be flat firmly on the floor, with a 90-degree angle on the legs.

The tips of the feet should be placed on the outside. The arms should be resting on the supports (where present) or on the thighs.

If there are supports, the hands should be left dangling.

If they are not present, the hands are resting on the legs, and the fingers are separate.

Position of the Coachman

This position allows you to be seated but without particular basic support. It can be practiced wherever you have something to sit on (a chair, a stone, a stool...).

You sit, for example, on the chair very far forward without leaning forward with your back.

Your feet must be flat firmly on the ground, with the tips pointing outwards. Your back should bend forward by resting your forearms on your thighs and letting your hands dangle between your legs so that they do not touch each other. Pivot your neck forward as much as possible, and relax your shoulders and jaw.

Other Suggestions

To achieve the best results, the environment must be quiet, the phone and any form of technological distraction must be disconnected beforehand. In the room, there must be a very soft light with a constant temperature that allows neither hot nor cold. The environmental conditions, in fact, influence our mood, and the acquisition of a correct position guarantees an objective relaxation of all the muscles.

Do not wear clothes that tighten and restrict your movement: for this purpose also remove the watch and glasses and loosen the belt.

It goes without saying that constancy is very important for achieving a psychic balance. It only takes 10 minutes a day, but a real reluctance is to be taken into consideration. Before doing this practice, you really need to give yourself some time. It must be a deliberate practice. This is one of the reasons why it is not advisable to practice it in small time gaps between commitments, but rather in dedicated time slots.

Also, it is advisable not to practice the exercises immediately after lunch to avoid sleep. At the end of each workout, perform awakening exercises except for the evening just before going to sleep.

At first, checking the relaxation of the various parts of the body will require some reflection. But over time and practice, everything will become more instinctive. Do not expect great results in the first days of practice. Do not abandon the practice immediately because, like anything else, you cannot expect to know how to do it immediately.

One last tip is to not be too picky when it comes to checking the position to take. In fact, the indications provided are broad; it is not necessary to interpret them rigidly.

Conclusion

Congratulations! You've now learned the basics of gastric band hypnosis and how to use it to empower yourself and strengthen the confidence in your ability to change habits and lose weight. Aside from biological and environmental, many psychological influences shape your thoughts, feelings, and behavioral patterns when it comes to eating.

Most people claim that weight loss hypnosis is a simple way to solve weight issues. People are also attracted by hypnosis because they feel they don't have to do any workouts, they can eat whatever they want, and all they have to do is close their eyes and lose weight in minutes. That's just not true.

No magic pills are available to lose weight, be it by hypnosis or some other form of weight loss. It is not possible to lose weight immediately after only one hypnosis session. A well-trained and professional hypnotist takes many sessions to achieve the best possible outcomes.

Several websites on the Internet say that weight loss hypnosis will produce dramatic results after just one session. Most people are likely to be insulted by this argument because everybody knows it is not possible to lose the weight overnight-however successful the hypnotist is.

Practicing weight loss hypnosis was another method for those who want to shape their bodies as they wish. There are also men who don't like their own body image. This leads to a loss of self-esteem and confidence. Some people prefer to use workouts and other lifestyle strategies to achieve their ideal body shape. Unfortunately, few tests are churning out. That is why people who understood the technique of mental strength resort to hypnosis to lose their body mass. You will find an absolute guide on how to use that method to attain the correct body shape on the internet. It is up to you to use your brain's strength to understand how useful it can be for you.

Hypnotizing is generally known to remove the inner self concentration. It generally happens in the same way as in a trance. Slimming hypnosis is an operation performed with the aid of the hypnotherapist. In this case, the person who wants to slightly repeat the messages given to him in the form of sentences, phrases, or even pictures may do so verbally. Mental images often play a major role in achieving the same result.

One thing you must remember is that your mind needs to concentrate more as you go through the hypnotizing process. In certain states, the mind and the subconscious state are very sensitive. You are well-positioned to react suggestively to the circumstances which lead you to your ideal body so that the best results can be obtained in a very short period of time. It is an activity that many people can do effectively with much less effort.

The research centers and interested stakeholders have performed many studies. Research has shown that people typically achieve fair outcomes using this form of hypnosis. This method can also lose up to an average of 2.7 kilograms.

Hypnotized, however, does not always function well on its own. You will take into account other behaviors that can effectively improve your weight loss. Take the best diet plan with your nutritionist's support. Not just this, you should do the workouts that will reduce your excess weight. In addition, you will try to follow a balanced lifestyle, which would help you in the end. Regulate your sleep hours, for example, and avoid any bad habits. If you use this routine and use all the tricks, you get the best performance. Ultimately, you learn to regulate your mind to lose weight. You train your subconscious mind to decrease your body mass, and if you practice this cycle, it will happen.